PSYCHOSOCIAL INTERVENTIONS IN HIV DISEASE

Cognitive-Behavioral Therapy

A book series edited by
Robert L. Russell, Ph.D.

This series presents the latest developments
in cognitive and cognitive-behavioral therapy.
The works in this series are written for practicing
cognitive-behavioral therapists as well as for psychodynamic
therapists who are eager to learn new ways of
understanding and helping their patients.

PSYCHOSOCIAL INTERVENTIONS IN HIV DISEASE

A Stage-Focused and Culture-Specific Approach

Edited by

Isiaah Crawford, Ph.D., and Baruch Fishman, Ph.D.

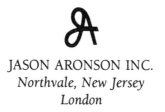

JASON ARONSON INC.
Northvale, New Jersey
London

Production Editor: M'lou Pinkham

This book was set in 11 pt. Berkeley Book by Alabama Book Composition of Deatsville, Alabama, and printed and bound by Book-mart Press, North Bergen, New Jersey.

Library of Congress Cataloging-in-Publication Data

Psychosocial interventions in HIV disease : a stage-focused and
  culture-specific approach / edited by Isiaah Crawford and Baruch
  Fishman.
        p. cm. — (Cognitive-behavioral therapy)
    Includes bibliographical references and index.
    ISBN 1-56821-825-7 (alk. paper)
    1. AIDS (Disease)—Patients—Mental health.   2. Cognitive therapy.
  3. Cultural psychiatry. I. Crawford, Isiaah. II. Fishman, Baruch.
  III. Series.
    [DNLM: 1. HIV Infections—psychology. 2. HIV Infections—therapy.
  3. Social Support.   WC 503.7 P974 1996]
  RC607.A26P7945 1996
  616.97′92′0019—dc20
  DNLM/DLC
  for Library of Congress   96-14097

Manufactured in the United States of America. Jason Aronson Inc. offers books and cassettes. For information and catalog write to Jason Aronson Inc., 230 Livingston Street, Northvale, New Jersey 07647.

Contents

Foreword

Increasingly, mental health professionals, including clinical psychologists, psychiatrists, and social workers, have been challenged to reorient their treatments to provide sensitive and effective interventions to those infected and affected by HIV disease. In truth, mental health professionals have been called to assist in the treatment and care of those afflicted by this illness. The call can take many forms, from devising and implementing stress-reduction interventions for those in the process of being tested for, or living with, HIV infection to preparing those in the late stages of the illness to deal with their own (and others') death(s). For the most part, even when the cause of HIV was unknown, this call has been responded to with compassion and improvisation on an individual basis. In a relatively brief period, this initial individual response has been transformed into scientific innovation in research and the growing availability of programmatic interventions organized at the community level.

Much still needs to be learned and accomplished, however. One ongoing task in need of immediate attention is to provide up-to-date information and instruction in therapeutic interventions to those providing frontline care, whether such care takes place in private practices, in out- or inpatient hospital units, or in the mental health centers that serve local communities. This volume provides the mental health practitioner with an innovative, frank, sensitive, and knowledgeable resource. It highlights up-to-date cognitive and cognitive-behavioral approaches as applied to the problems associated with HIV illness. In fact, the mental health practitioner is offered not only a concise overview of the history, epidemiology, and clinical course of HIV disease in the United States, but discussion and illustration of interventions designed to prevent high-risk behaviors, maximize quality and quantity of life for those living with HIV disease, and augment coping strategies for those faced with impending death.

In addition, however, what makes this volume distinct is its sensitivity to the specific challenges that each stage of HIV infection presents and to how sociocultural contexts and ethnic identity shape some of the cognitive and behavioral responses individuals have toward HIV and their illness. Mental health professionals will find chapters that focus on interventions with African-American and Hispanic gay and bisexual men as well as chapters devoted to issues concerning women and HIV and injection drug users and HIV. Importantly for a volume that hopes to augment the actual clinical skills of mental health practitioners, many of the chapters include specific treatment recommendations and case vignettes to illustrate intervention strategies and concrete techniques.

Adding to the clinical strength of this volume is the level of experience and involvement the authors have had in their own clinical practices or treatment research with individuals struggling with HIV. These are not chapters written "from afar," but by consummate professionals who have devoted a great deal of their work-life trying to prevent and alleviate the suffering that HIV disease can cause. Consequently, the mental health practitioner is invited to consider in the frankest terms frontline problems and innovative problem-solving procedures, backed by research where possible, to deal with them. Anyone who is in clinical practice will undoubtably benefit from the experience and scholarly reflection distilled in this book. In fact, without hyperbole, I can say that it is my expectation that the serious consideration of this volume will change and/or augment how clinicians engage HIV-infected or -affected individuals and, if not outright save, then surely enrich, their clients' lives.

—*Robert L. Russell*

Preface

The physical, emotional, and financial devastation caused by AIDS is now well into its second decade. Since its discovery in 1981 (Centers for Disease Control and Prevention [CDC] 1981), AIDS has spread at an epidemic rate in the United States and throughout the world (Shubert 1992). A great deal has been learned about AIDS over this fifteen-year period. HIV, the causative agent for AIDS, has been identified (Barre-Sinoussi et al. 1983), along with assessment procedures to detect laboratory evidence of its presence (i.e., HIV antibody testing); medical management strategies and drug treatments have been established; and numerous prevention and health promotion campaigns have been implemented throughout the world. Although biomedical scientists are vigorously pursuing the development of an AIDS vaccine or cure, the outgrowth of these efforts is many years away and health care providers will have to continue to address the challenges presented by HIV/AIDS.

Although many social scientists have been intricately involved in designing and implementing HIV/AIDS education, therapeutic, and behavior change programs, the limited amount of research available (Crawford et al. 1991, Dhooper et al. 1987–1988, Knox et al. 1989, Trezza 1994) indicates that most mental health professionals do not gather systematic training in HIV/AIDS issues, continue to have significant knowledge deficits about HIV, and have biases against persons living with AIDS. As the AIDS pandemic continues to rage forward, mental health professionals will be encountering individuals affected by HIV in their clinical practices; consequently, it is imperative for them to be well informed about the disease and its treatment.

HIV infection is a chronic, multistage illness that progresses from an emotionally challenging asymptomatic stage to physically deteriorating and ultimately fatal stages over several years. Over the course of the illness, patients experience multiple challenges that can be unique to the stage of their illness, gender, sexual orientation, or ethnic/racial background. These challenges require flexible and effective coping skills, both specialized and general, in order to manage the emotional, behavioral, and interpersonal disturbances that often accompany HIV illness.

Patients at every stage of HIV infection need effective and focused educational and psychosocial interventions to help them cope and adjust to their illness. But because of the unique and variable characteristics of the illness, and the patients afflicted, there is no one universal intervention that is always appropriate. The challenges of enhancing cooperation with medical treatment, modifying risky behaviors, and alleviating suffering among the diverse populations impacted by HIV require specialized expertise and the adoption of general psychological-educational interventions. Over the last few years, several interventions of this kind have been designed, developed, and successfully tested. This book describes them in detail; the following introductory chapter provides a general background and outline.

REFERENCES

Barre-Sinoussi, F., Chermann, J. C., Rey, F., et al. (1983). Isolation of a t-lymphotropic retrovirus from a patient at risk for acquired immune-deficiency syndrome (AIDS): *Science* 220: 868–871.

Centers for Disease Control and Prevention (1981). Pneumocystis peneumonia: Los Angeles. *Morbidity and Mortality Weekly Report* 30:250–252.

Crawford, I., Humfleet, G., Ribordy, S., et al. (1991). Stigmatization of AIDS patients by mental health professionals. *Professional Psychology: Research and Practice* 22:357–361.

Dhooper, S. S., Royse, D. D., and Tran, T. V. (1987–1988). Social work practitioners' attitudes towards AIDS victims. *Journal of Applied Social Sciences* 12:108–123.

Knox, M. D., Dow, M. G., and Cotton, D. A. (1989). Mental health care providers: the need for AIDS education. *AIDS Education & Prevention* 1:285–290.

Shubert, V. (1992). Introduction. In *AIDS Crisis in America: A Reference Handbook: Contemporary World Issues*, ed. M. E. Hombs. Santa Barbara, CA: ABC–CLIO.

Trezza, G. R. (1994). HIV knowledge and stigmatization of persons with AIDS: implications for the development of HIV education for young adults. *Professional Psychology: Research and Practice* 25:141–148.

About the Editors

Dr. Isiaah Crawford is an associate professor in the Department of Psychology at Loyola University Chicago. He completed his doctorate in clinical psychology at DePaul University in 1987. He maintains an active private practice, specializing in the treatment of individuals living with HIV disease, depression, and addictive behaviors. He has published in the areas of HIV prevention, human sexuality, and professional practice and training.

Dr. Baruch Fishman is the director of the Cognitive Psychotherapy Training Program and Clinic at the Department of Psychiatry, New York Hospital-Cornell Medical Center. He received his Ph.D. in experimental and clinical psychology from the University of Pennsylvania in 1984, and has published articles on the use of cognitive-behavioral therapy with depressed HIV-infected patients and for pain management.

Acknowledgments

We would like to express our gratitude to the contributing authors of this book. Without their commitment and steadfast efforts this volume would not have been possible. All of the chapters were formulated with great care and clearly demonstrate the scholarship and clinical expertise of the authors.

We would also like to thank Robert L. Russell, Ph.D., for his support and encouragement throughout all phases of this project. His clear and unwavering belief in the importance of the book and the contribution it would make to the field was inspirational.

There are numerous technical tasks to be performed in constructing a book of this nature. We owe a debt of gratitude to Dorothy Morgan for her assistance in producing the book and for the many services she performed to help bring the project to fruition. In addition, we want to thank Jason Aronson Inc. and its publisher, Michael Moskowitz, Ph.D., for their enthusiasm and support for this publication. The compassionate and skillful technical editing services provided by M'lou Pinkham were invaluable and enhanced the quality of the text.

This book is dedicated to the memory of Samuel Perry, M.D., professor of psychiatry at Cornell University Medical College, a pioneer in the study and treatment of emotional distress in patients with HIV/AIDS. He was a mentor and continues to be a source of inspiration for Baruch Fishman, Ph.D. The book is also dedicated to the memory of Arthurine K. Crawford. Her numerous sacrifices and devotion to Isiaah Crawford, Ph.D., continue to sustain and motivate him.

Contributors

Isiaah Crawford, Ph.D.
Loyola University Chicago

Baruch Fishman, Ph.D.
Cornell University Medical College, New York, New York

Ralph J. DiClemente, Ph.D.
School of Public Health Behavior,
University of Alabama, Birmingham

Catherine M. Flanagan, Ph.D.
Cornell University Medical College, New York, New York

Vicki Gluhoski, Ph.D.
Cornell University Medical College, New York, New York

Andrea Hamilton
Northwestern University Medical School, Chicago, Illinois

Denise Hornbuckle, Ed.D.
Substance Abuse Treatment Programs,
University of Alabama, Birmingham

Norman Huggins, M.D.
Center for AIDS Research, University of Alabama, Birmingham

Gary Humfleet, Ph.D.
San Francisco Veterans Administration Medical Center

Catherine Leake
Loyola University Chicago

Shandowyn L. Parker, MPH
School of Medicine, Department of Pediatrics
Division of General Pediatrics & Adolescent Medicine
University of Alabama, Birmingham

Doreen Salina, Ph.D.
Northwestern University Medical School, Chicago, Illinois

Tomas Soto, Ph.D.
Cook County Hospital, Chicago, Illinois

An Introduction to HIV Infection: Its History, Virology, and Biopsychosocial Stages

BARUCH FISHMAN AND ISIAAH CRAWFORD

HISTORY AND EPIDEMIOLOGY

Acquired immunodeficiency syndrome was first identified in the United States in 1981. Physicians in New York City and San Francisco began to encounter the death of a growing number of men who developed illnesses that are normally warded off by the body's natural defenses. The causative agent for these deaths was eventually determined to be a virus, the human immunodeficiency virus (HIV). There is evidence from frozen stored blood samples that the virus was infecting these men at least as early as 1978 (Centers for Disease Control and Prevention [CDC] 1987). Since that time, the total number of reported cases of AIDS has risen to 476,899 in this country alone (CDC 1995). The World Health Organization also estimates that at least one million Americans are currently infected with HIV, most of whom will develop related illnesses in the next ten years (WHO 1992). The incidence of AIDS doubled every six months during the early years of the epidemic; currently, it doubles every sixteen to eighteen months (CDC 1993). AIDS is the leading cause of death for young men and women between the ages of 25 and 34 years in the United States.

WHO estimates that at least nine to eleven million adults have been infected and one million children have been born infected with the virus. Most of the individuals living with AIDS are in the sub-Saharan region of Africa, and Asia is poised to become the next AIDS epicenter. WHO reports that the pattern of transmission of HIV in these regions of the world is primarily through hetero-sexual contact and the male-to-female ratio is approximately 1:1.

In the United States AIDS has had the greatest impact upon the gay and bisexual male population; the face of the epidemic is changing, however. As of June 1995, the CDC reported that of the total number of AIDS cases, 244,235 (52 percent) were reportedly the result of men having sex with men; 118,694 (25 percent) were attributed to intravenous (IV) drug use; and 35,683 (8 percent) were attributed to heterosexual transmission. The Bureau of the Census (1993) reports that African-Americans and Hispanics account for 12 and 9 percent, respectively, of the United States pop-ulation; however, they account for 48 percent of the cases of AIDS in this country. Chapters 5 and 6 of this book discuss the factors underlying these findings, along with psychotherapeutic and prevention strategies salient to individuals in these communities.

The rate of HIV infection has leveled off in the adult gay community in the United States as a result of effective prevention programs. Unfortunately, infection rates have increased steadily among IV drug users, women, and adolescents. In fact, newly reported AIDS cases among IV drug users outnumber those among gay and bisexual men (Shubert 1992). Women account for the fastest growing category of cases: from 1991 to 1992 there was a 35 percent increase in the number of women diagnosed with AIDS. Women with AIDS are overwhelmingly African-American (53 percent) or Hispanic (21 percent), and 79 percent of pediatric AIDS cases are African-American and Hispanic (CDC 1993). Chapters 7 and 8 elaborate on the distinctive treatment and health promotion issues relevant to women and injection drug users who are confronted with the realities of HIV.

What is HIV?

HIV is a retrovirus, which means that its genetic material is not deoxyribonucleic acid (DNA) but ribonucleic acid (RNA). The retrovirus label stems from the enzyme that allows HIV to replicate—reverse transcriptase. This allows the virus to insert itself into the DNA of CD-4 (Cluster Determinant; previously called T4) cells in the immune system (Batchelor 1988). The immune system responds to HIV as it does to other viruses that invade the body, by producing antibodies in an effort to prevent infection; due to the unique nature of HIV, however, the immune system response is unable to reach the virus that integrates itself into the CD-4 cells' DNA, and these infected cells remain untouched and the virus multiplies. Over time, more and more of the CD-4 cells are killed or rendered ineffective by HIV; eventually this deficit begins to impair not only the ability of the immune system to fight off infections by viruses and other parasitic organisms, but its ability to detect and destroy mutated cancer cells. At this stage the individual begins to be affected by a large variety of opportunistic infections and cancers that eventually lead to death.

Although there is not yet a cure for HIV infection—in the sense of killing all of the HIV in the body—several drugs slow its replication and the loss of CD-4 cells, and there are many improved treatments for the more common infections and cancers. In addition, some of the common infections can actually be prevented by the use of chronic, prophylactic antibiotics. For example, Pneumocystis carinii pneumonia, a particularly lethal form of pneumonia, used to be a major cause of death early in the epidemic, but has become much less prevalent in recent years because most HIV-infected patients with impaired immune function take preventive antibiotics regularly.

BIOPSYCHOSOCIAL STAGES OF HIV INFECTION

Biological/Medical Stages

From the biological or medical perspective, the course of HIV infection is often viewed in four stages:

1. *Acute/Primary HIV Disease* occurs shortly after the initial infection with HIV. It is a mild illness lasting up to two weeks with nonspecific symptoms similar to mononucleosis and other mild, self-limited infections. As a consequence of this illness, specific antibodies for HIV develop over a period of six weeks to six months. These antibodies circulate in the blood of an infected person and can be detected with widely available laboratory tests. At the primary stage of HIV infection, however, there are no HIV antibodies in the blood yet and therefore no routine way to determine a diagnosis. Only specialized and rather expensive laboratory tests that detect the actual presence of specific HIV proteins can provide a definitive diagnosis. This condition is thus rarely reported by patients or recognized by physicians.

2. *Chronic Asymptomatic HIV Disease* can last many years and involves no noticeable bodily symptoms. During this period, patients may or may not know that they are infected with HIV, and if they do know they may or may not take prophylactic medications. Over the years, in this stage, the immune system is slowly damaged by HIV, mostly by killing CD-4 lymphocytes. When the number of CD-4 cells falls below 200–300 cells/microliter (from above 700 cells/microliter normally), chronic physical symptoms of the third stage appear.

3. *Chronic Symptomatic HIV Disease* is marked by a variety of illness manifestations that can be mild to

moderate in intensity. As the number of CD-4 cells drops, the most common set of symptoms to develop is labeled "constitutional": fever, night sweats, reduced appetite, fatigue, and weight loss. Often there is swelling and pain in several lymph nodes, and a large variety of minor, but irritating, so-called "opportunistic infections." These include itchy skin due to folliculitis, herpes-zoster (shingles), canker sores, oral thrush, and vaginal candidiasis, among many others. Many of these minor infections can be treated effectively and most patients who receive medical treatment also begin to take prophylactic antibiotics and antiviral medications such as AZT. This stage can also last several years, but eventually most patients progress to the most advanced HIV disease.

4. *Advanced HIV Disease/AIDS* involves severely deteriorating physical and mental functioning, ultimately leading to death. At this stage the immune system is almost completely ineffective in protecting the body and very serious opportunistic infections and cancers systematically destroy various organ systems. Most commonly affected are the skin and other mucous membranes, the gastrointestinal tract, the brain, the lungs, and the lymphatic system. As a result of numerous advances in the diagnosis and treatment of most of these conditions, patients do live longer and with better quality of life before the body is overwhelmed.

HIV infects the cells of the immune system by gaining entry into the bloodstream in the following ways: unprotected sexual contact, sharing of injection drug equipment among infected persons, transfusion of infected blood or blood products, and congenital or perinatal transmission from a woman to her fetus or newborn (CDC 1994). HIV cannot be transmitted through routine, nonsexual contact that occurs in the home, office, or classroom (Koop 1986).

The presence of HIV infection may be detected by culturing the virus, identifying viral proteins or genetic material, and measuring antibodies produced against the virus (Glasner and Kaslow 1990). At present, the diagnosis of HIV infection is rendered primarily from tests determining the presence of HIV antibodies, which can be detected six weeks to three months after HIV infection. Although no diagnostic test is completely accurate, the recommended HIV serologic testing sequence has been shown to be highly reliable (Sloand et al. 1991).

PSYCHOSOCIAL STAGES OF HIV INFECTION

The biological/medical perspective in the case of HIV disease does not directly describe the psychological experience of the patient: the patient, as a person, exists in subjective, interpersonal, and social contexts that precede the infection and affect the actual experience of each individual in unique ways. However, since the medical challenges are common for most patients, a four-stage process can be conceptualized:

1. Pre-HIV antibody testing: possibility of being infected
2. Post-HIV antibody testing: knowledge of being seroposi- tive, asymptomatic, stable CD-4 count
3. Falling CD-4 count: with or without physical symptoms and/or prophylactic medications
4. Severe medical illness: AIDS, deteriorating physical and mental functioning, pending and eventual death

Each stage can actually involve several challenges or stressors that vary in particular individuals, but the underlying emotional challenges are similar across individuals and stages of illness. The intensity of emotional challenges increases with the progression from stage to stage for all patients, but clinical experience and research findings indicate that many patients cope well with the distress associated with their illness and go through this process without excessive emotional, behavioral, or interpersonal disturbances. On the other hand, a substantial proportion, estimated at 15 to 20 percent of the patients, do manifest such disturbances. These patients, like less distressed individuals, face a challenging medical reality that they realistically interpret as threatening; in contrast to those who cope well, however, emotionally distressed patients believe they are extremely vulnerable, and feel unequipped, helpless, and hopeless in coping with the challenge of their illness. In vulnerable individuals the presence of thinking distortions, misinterpretations, and a sense of poor personal control combine with bodily symptoms of anxiety, depression, and anger to produce chronically escalating distress.

The specific challenges faced by HIV-infected patients range from uncertainty and disruption of social relations to coping with disease symptoms and aggressive treatments while tolerating the frustration of personal and interpersonal needs and aspirations. When there are even minor physical symptoms for a long period this challenge becomes still harder. The constant or fluctuating presence of fatigue, sweating, nausea, and other pains and aches in consciousness can disrupt normal mental processes and personal activities.

This chronic experience can be described along the emotional dimensions of *confusion, anxiety, anger,* and *sadness.* Such emotional reactions occur, at times, in most chronic, life-threatening illnesses (e.g., cancer, heart disease, diabetes), and often the presence of noxious sensory impulses (i.e., somatic symptoms) becomes the focused stressor because it serves as a constant reminder of the patient's condition.

CONFUSION.   Some degree of confusion is almost always present in patients with HIV infection, and on occasion this state can become severe enough to require psychiatric or other medical interventions. The term *confusion* refers to a state of disorientation and disorganization of normal mental processes that can be caused by psychological and/or organic disturbances. Confusion is generally associated with some degree of emotional distress; shortened attention span; impairments of concentration, memory, and comprehension; and a weakened sense of personal control. The psychological pressures experienced by HIV-infected patients are numerous. These stressors often include the bombardment of sometimes conflictual medical information, multiple hospitalizations, the need to make critical medical decisions, and other disruption of normal daily routines and social relations. Numerous organic causes can be present and some are listed below. Severe confusion can be caused by the following conditions:

Psychological	Organic
Severe psychopathology	HIV-related dementia
Intense emotional experiences	Drug intoxication
Stressful medical treatments and diagnostic procedures	Medication side effects and complications
Medical decisions under uncertainty	Metabolic abnormalities
Conflicting information about AIDS	Severe intractable pain
Disruption of social relations	
Disruption of daily routine	

ANXIETY.   The emotional arousal experienced as anxiety is generally associated with the perception of threat, or the anticipation of impending harm to the self. In the case of HIV infection, persistent cues from family, friends, and the media, as well as the knowledge of HIV infection or the presence of somatic symptoms, continue to remind patients of the multiple threats and potential harms that are associated with their condition at every stage of HIV disease. Individuals may focus on different aspects of danger, but all HIV-infected patients share the most anxiety-provoking condition of living: *general uncertainty*. Some of the specific threats to personal integrity commonly perceived by HIV-infected patients include:

Medical and Physical Threats	Personal and Social Threats
Chronic disturbing symptoms	Loss of dignity (self-control)
Reinoculation	Loss of mental abilities
Disfigurement	Loss of social status
Physical disability	Loss of employment
Treatment failure	Financial loss
Uncontrollable pain	Loss of independence
Advancing disease	Harm to family/friends
Death	Stigmatization, rejection
	Exposure of intimate secrets
	Infecting sexual partners with HIV

ANGER   From the time of seropositive notification, and throughout the course of the illness, patients may experience various degrees of anger. Anger in general is associated with the perception of a destructive attack on the person and/or frustration of goals and aspirations. Many situations may trigger angry reactions in HIV-infected patients, from the appearance of unpleasant symptoms to personal and economic losses. In fact, any of the conditions mentioned before as potential threats that provoke anxiety can trigger anger when it is about to happen or when it actually happens. Normally, angry arousal is triggered fast and dissipates quickly when frustration is resolved, but when threats and frustrations are persistent, angry arousal can become chronic and mounting. Chronic anger can complicate the medical management of HIV-infected patients because it is associated with chronic autonomic mobilization and bodily tension. Chronic anger can also interfere with the patient's social relations because it is associated with increased irritability, reduced frustration tolerance, poor cooperation, a hostile attitude, and impulsive-aggressive action.

SADNESS.   When any of the potential threats mentioned above becomes a reality and is perceived as a permanent loss in the domain of the self, the emotion of sadness is experienced. Sadness and grief, natural and adaptive reactions to appraisal of loss, diminish over time. But when the appraisal of specific losses is overgeneralized by the patient to all aspects of the personal domain, and/or when the specific loss affects appraisals of personal worth, dignity, and identity, a sense of humiliation and self-rejection may produce the pathological condition of depression. Depression is associated with physiological disturbances (e.g., loss of appetite and libido, sleep disturbance), cognitive causes (e.g., distorted thinking, loss of hope, loss of self-esteem), and affective-motivational changes (e.g., crying, helplessness, disinterest, social withdrawal). As is the case with chronic anxiety and anger, depression can compromise both the medical and the psychosocial conditions of patients.

At any time during the course of their illness, HIV-infected patients may experience any or several of the emotional states described above in the context of general confusion. Patients may feel the sadness associated with the reality of the losses they have already incurred, anxiety about their uncertain condition and the potential of additional harms, and anger about the frustration of their aspirations and the harm they suffer. As time goes on in chronic stress, even normally adjusted individuals and well-functioning social support systems (family, friends, lovers) may be slowly worn down and experience deterioration in coping efforts and well-being. The patient may then feel more confused, isolated, anxious, and angry or sad. Since increasing emotional distress is associated with growing frustration and symptom intolerance, losses and symptoms are experienced as intensifying and treatment is experienced as failing. This further distresses the patient and his support system and increases overall suffering. Chapters 3 through 8 outline in greater detail the emotional course of HIV disease and treatment recommendations for the mental health professional to consider in his or her work with HIV-impacted people.

DIVERSITY AND HIV

Unlike many aspects of contemporary society, HIV is not particularly discriminating. Its impact crosses the boundaries of gender, race, culture, socioeconomic status, sexual orientation, age, and religion. Attempting to conceptualize the biopsychosocial effect of HIV with one comprehensive model, like the one previously described, is naive and foolhardy. Although having a basic framework to understand the myriad medical and psychological phenomena that takes place with individuals infected with HIV is helpful, one must acknowledge the unique interplay of HIV with the culture, race, gender, and sexual orientation of the person affected by the virus. Assisting the reader in recognizing when and how models of this nature should be used, how medical and psychological stages vary across races and cultures, and how treatment strategies should be tailored to the specific needs of HIV-impacted people are the primary goals of this book. It is our belief that the subsequent chapters will provide the reader with the information and skills necessary to provide effective culture-specific mental health care to people impacted by HIV.

REFERENCES

Batchelor, W. (1988). AIDS 1988: the science and the limits of science. *American Psychologist* 43:853–858.

Bureau of the Census (1993). *Statistical Abstracts of the United States*, 113th ed. Washington, DC: U.S. Government Printing Office.

Centers for Disease Control and Prevention (CDC). (1987). Revision of the CDC surveillance case definition for AIDS. *Morbidity and Mortality Weekly Report* 35:669–671.

Centers for Disease Control and Prevention. (1993). *HIV/AIDS Surveillance Report*, 5(4). Atlanta: U.S. Department of Health and Human Services.

Centers for Disease Control and Prevention. (1994). *HIV/AIDS Surveillance Report*, 6(2). Atlanta: U.S. Department of Health and Human Services.

Centers for Disease Control and Prevention. (1995). *HIV/AIDS Surveillance Report*, 7(1). Atlanta: U.S. Department of Health and Human Services.

Glasner, P. D., and Kaslow, R. A. (1990). The epidemiology of human immunodeficiency virus infection. *Journal of Consulting and Clinical Psychology* 58:13–21.

Koop, C. E. (1986). *The Surgeon General's report on acquired immune deficiency syndrome*. Washington, DC: U.S. Government Printing Office.

Shubert, V. (1992). Introduction: In *AIDS Crisis in America: A Reference Handbook: Contemporary World Issues*, ed. M. E. Hombs. Santa Barbara, CA: ABC–CLIO.

Sloand, E., Pitt, E., Chiarello, R., and Nemo, G. (1991). HIV testing: state of the art. *Journal of the American Medical Association*, 266:2861–2866.

World Health Organization (1992). *Current and future dimensions of the HIV/AIDS pandemic*. Washington, DC: World Health Organization.

2

Integrating Safer-Sex Training Into Psychotherapy

GARY HUMFLEET

As described in Chapter 1, HIV is transmitted from one individual to another through the exchange of bodily fluids. To be at risk for HIV infection two individuals must exchange blood, semen, vaginal fluids, or urine during sexual activities. Since no vaccine or cure for HIV infection appears imminent, it is critical that people learn to reduce their risks for transmission of this virus and protect themselves from initial, as well as repeated, infections with HIV. Safer sex is an important issue for seropositive as well as seronegative individuals. Different strains of HIV exist and their relative impact on the body may vary (Levy 1993). Experts believe exposure to additional HIV may accelerate the impact of the infection on the immune system by introducing more virulent strains of the virus. Therefore, it is important for seropositive individuals to protect themselves from reinfection with HIV. In addition, seropositive individuals need to protect themselves from other sexually transmitted infections, such as hepatitis. With a compromised immune system, the body is less able to fight these and other infections. Mental health professionals in the 1990s have a responsibility to educate clients about HIV risks, assist them in identifying barriers to risk reduction, and work with them to develop and implement alternative behaviors.

With what type of client should a therapist discuss safer sex? Historically, much of the discussion about transmission of HIV has focused on *risk groups* (e.g., injection drug users, homosexuals, hemophiliacs, prostitutes). As a psychotherapist, it is important to think in terms of *risk behavior* rather than *risk groups*. Sexually active individuals cannot be absolutely certain of their partner's sex or drug-use history. For example, a young, heterosexual woman may engage in anal sex with her boyfriend. From their point of view, this behavior allows sexual expression while maintaining the young woman's "virginity." However, if the male partner occasionally injects drugs or engages in homosexual behavior, a member of a relatively lower risk group (the young woman) is engaging in a high-risk behavior. It is imperative that detailed sexual behavior and drug-use histories and discussion of safer sexual activities be considered with all sexually active clients. In order to do this competently, it is important to know the variety of sexual behaviors practiced by individuals and their associated risks for HIV infection.

WHAT IS SAFER SEX?

Sexual behaviors can be placed on a continuum in terms of risks for HIV transmission. For the purposes of this chapter, the continuum has been divided into three general risk levels (Table 2–1): behaviors considered *safe*, behaviors considered *less safe*, and behaviors considered *unsafe*.

TABLE 2-1

Considered Safe

Solo masturbation
Mutual masturbation
Dry kissing
Use of sexual toys (without sharing)
Hugging
Frottage (Body rubbing)
Massage
Light sadomasochism (without bleeding or bruising)

Considered Less Safe

Wet kissing
Oral sex (penile, vaginal, or anal) with a condom or latex barrier
(used correctly)
Anal sex with a condom
Vaginal sex with a condom
Water sports (external)
Fisting with gloves

Considered Unsafe

Oral sex (penile, vaginal, or anal) without a condom
Anal sex without a condom
Vaginal sex without a condom
Water sports (internal) or broken skin
Sharing sex toys
Fisting

Behaviors Considered Safe

In general, sexual choices that provide no risk of HIV transmission are those that prohibit the exchange of bodily fluids: semen, vaginal secretions, blood, urine, or feces. This category includes activities performed alone or with a partner, all of which can be enhanced through the use of fantasy, talking, and visual stimuli (e.g., videos). As you can see from Table 2–1, these activities do not involve penetration by either partner. However, they may include contact of bodily fluids from one partner with the skin of the other partner. Intact skin serves as an excellent barrier to the transmission of HIV as well as other viruses or bacteria. Hence, the safer sex slogan used by many HIV educators: "On me, not in me." The only concern for transmission in these cases is when the skin is not intact due to open lesions or cuts.

Although not specifically included on the list, abstinence from sexual activities falls within this class of risk-reduction methods. When discussing options for reducing the risk of HIV infection, a client may choose, or a therapist may recommend, abstinence. This can be a valid choice for a client, but it does not preclude the need for education and information about safer sexual practices. It has been my clinical experience that some clients choose abstinence as a risk-reduction technique either on their own (e.g., in response to fear) or on the recommendations of others. These clients struggle with that choice, frequently relapsing to sexual activities. Although there is no intention to have sexual contact, the client may impulsively engage in sex and not be prepared to protect him- or herself. For example, a client who has chosen abstinence as a risk-reduction method may not have considered the steps involved in negotiating safer sex with a partner. If this individual does engage in sex, attempts at safer sex negotiations are likely to fail.

Behaviors Considered Less Safe

This category includes behaviors that pose minimal risk for transmission as well as those that incorporate barriers that prevent the exchange of body fluids. Wet kissing is considered a minimal-risk behavior because the concentration of HIV in saliva is not thought to be sufficient for HIV transmission. Any concern about wet kissing is due to the possible exchange of blood; however, no cases of HIV infection by this route have been identified. To be considered safer than unsafe, barriers must be *used correctly* and *remain intact*. A condom used for anal or vaginal intercourse must be put on correctly with a water-based lubricant to reduce the possibility of breakage. The penis must be erect during withdrawal and the condom must be held at the base and removed away from the partner to prevent spillage of semen. If the condom breaks during sexual activities, the individual may be at a higher risk for HIV infection.

Behaviors Considered Unsafe

This category includes behaviors that frequently result in the exchange of bodily fluids. Engaging in these activities without the use of a barrier must be considered risky. One behavior that has posed difficulties for educators is oral sex. Early in the HIV epidemic there were no identified cases of HIV infection through oral sex. More recently, however, cases of HIV infection as a result of fellatio with ejaculation in the mouth have been reported (e.g., Lifson et al. 1990). A risk behavior that remains somewhat controversial is fellatio with withdrawal prior to ejaculation. Two factors need to be considered when educating clients. Prior to ejaculation, the release of small amounts of semen (pre-ejaculate) have the potential to reach the bloodstream of the receptive partner, resulting in HIV infection. Second, although withdrawal before ejaculation may be intended, this effort may not be successful. For these reasons, withdrawal prior to ejaculation during oral, as well as vaginal and anal, sex cannot be recommended as a safer sexual activity.

PSYCHOSOCIAL ISSUES RELATED TO UNSAFE SEX

Many studies have demonstrated that having accurate HIV knowledge does not necessarily lead to a reduction in risk behaviors (Kelly et al. 1993, Zimmerman and Olson 1994). Additional research has examined the correlates of high-risk behaviors. A therapist cannot effectively integrate risk-reduction training into treatment without understanding the factors relating to and needs being met through sex. For the purposes of this presentation, these issues are divided into two areas, situational factors and psychological factors.

Situational Factors

When working to reduce high-risk behaviors, clients often report personal, interpersonal, or social variables that interfere with their ability to engage in safer sexual relations. It is not unusual for clients to complain about condom use. Frequently they state that they or their partners are resistant because condoms decrease pleasure, are uncomfortable, and/or interfere with the spontaneity of sexual relations. When working with such clients, it is important to begin by acknowledging that condoms do decrease sensitivity. Next, the therapist should explore the client's feelings about condoms, and assist him or her in thinking of ways to integrate condoms into sex without disrupting the pleasurable aspects of sexuality.

Some individuals report difficulties with risk reduction because the sexual encounter was unplanned and they were not prepared. Making changes and reducing one's risk for HIV infection is easier if the environment is prepared to support low-risk behaviors. Many sexually active clients can prepare their environments by making a list of supplies—condoms, dental dams, water-based lubricants—and ensuring that they are available. A travel kit might help to ensure that risk reduction can occur outside the home.

A major factor that impacts one's ability to reduce risk successfully is discomfort or difficulty in talking directly to a partner about sex. Many people find it difficult to communicate their sexual desires and needs to their partner(s). For years, sex therapists have advocated verbal communication between partners to increase pleasure and sexual gratification. However, people continue to be reluctant to express what they like or dislike. With some of these individuals, therapists merely need to reassure them that talking about sex is okay and then discuss mechanisms to practice and introduce negotiation strategies into their sex lives. For others, a reluctance to talk with partners may be exacerbated by previous experiences or emotions. Some clients are reluctant to introduce safer sexual techniques due to fear of offending, and ultimately being rejected by, a partner. Others may perceive the introduction of safer activities as indicative of a lack of trust between partners. Yet others may have experienced sexual abuse or trauma that inhibits direct communication in these situations.

Psychological Factors

In addition to situational variables that play into unsafe sexual relations, psychological factors can influence the likelihood of initiating and maintaining safer sexual relationships. Many of these factors apply to both seronegative and seropositive individuals. Issues specific to seropositive or seronegative individuals are noted below.

The Meaning of Sex

The meaning of sex and sexual activities in a person's life strongly influences the ability to change sexual behaviors. For many individuals, particularly gay men, sexuality and sexual behavior is closely tied to self-identity. For gay men, sexual behaviors are closely tied to the development of a gay identity. Sexual behaviors are often an integral part of the coming-out process and remain a core aspect of a positive gay self-image. Sex functions as a way of expressing and affirming one's identity. Sex may also be a key step in starting a relationship. For some young adults, having sexual intercourse with a number of partners boosts not only their self-image but their status among peers. Regardless of sexual orientation, sex may be a way to obtain intimacy and express emotions. For many individuals the exchange of bodily fluids during sex is often an expression of the intimacy in the relationship, signifying that this partner is "special." By practicing safer sex, an individual may feel a loss of part of his or her identity or a critical intimate aspect of a relationship.

Denial

Although educated about HIV transmission and risk behaviors, some clients may continue to engage in high-risk sexual and drug activities while denying the risk. Denial can take many forms. Some individuals engage in unsafe sex and deny the risk of that specific incident. For example, a client may perceive an unsafe sexual act as less risky because the partner was familiar or didn't "look" sick or infected. In a study I coordinated in the Los Angeles area targeting men who have sex with men but do not identify as gay, we found that many of these men did not believe they were at risk. Some individuals engaging in risky behaviors felt they were not at risk simply because they were not gay, regardless of their sexual behavior. Others felt that since they were the insertive partners, they were also not at risk. Denial may also be a significant factor for individuals who engage in high-risk behavior and remain seronegative, particularly if they know their partner is seropositive. This individual may deny the risk by believing he or she is somehow immune to HIV infection: "If I don't have it by now, I'll never get it." Due to this denial, unsafe sex may continue.

A form of denial that is relevant for adolescents and young adults is their sense of invulnerability at this stage of life: they commonly believe they are not susceptible to a variety of life's dangers. Although this is a normal stage of development, it can become dangerous when considered in the context of HIV. It is not unusual for adolescents and young adults to perceive HIV as a problem for the older generation, something that can't happen to them. This attitude may contribute to the recent findings by some researchers, for example, Hays and colleagues (1990), that unprotected sex and HIV infection rates among younger gay men have increased.

Self-Esteem

A poor level of self-esteem, decreasing the individual's desire to consider safer sexual activities, may contribute to the likelihood of unsafe sex: he or she may not feel worth protecting. In addition, a poor self-image can affect the individual's ability to carry out risk-reduction efforts. Without a positive sense of self-worth, an individual may not feel a sense of control in sexual situations and may be reluctant to actively negotiate safer sex. Another factor that may contribute to self-esteem issues for a gay client is internalized homophobia. Historically, gay and lesbian individuals have been feared, hated, perceived as sick or evil, and discriminated against. Many gays and lesbians struggle with these societal attitudes, often leading to a poor self-image. Since the beginning of the epidemic, HIV disease has also carried a stigma. It is not unusual for gays and lesbians to hear from community, and sometimes family, members that HIV is a punishment for sick or sinful behaviors. Some individuals internalize these beliefs, feeling bad about themselves and who they are. In extreme situations individuals may believe they deserve to die, and thus continue to engage in high-risk behaviors.

Depression

Depression can impact risk-reduction efforts in several ways. For the seropositive client, depression may be acted out as a desire not to survive. "What difference does it make? I am going to die anyway. The sooner, the better." Such statements exemplify this affective state. For others, sex may be a method of coping with unresolved grief or sadness resulting from previous losses. Regardless of its origin, depression is often accompanied by feelings of hopelessness and helplessness. Those feelings can significantly interfere with efforts to protect oneself from HIV infection.

Survivor Guilt

Given the magnitude of deaths and losses since the beginning of the AIDS epidemic, it is not unusual for individuals to experience survivor guilt. Many people have felt the impact of HIV throughout their lives and their social networks. These individuals may serve, or have served, as a caretaker for friends, lovers, and/or family members with AIDS. They may have experienced numerous losses, may perceive their own risk for HIV as being similar to others in their life, and may begin to question why they are not dying. This may result in feelings of guilt and anxiety about surviving, possibly raising questions about their own self-worth. This is particularly true for seronegative individuals, although it can happen with long-term asymptomatic seropositives. Some of these individuals may cope with this guilt and anxiety by engaging in high-risk behaviors. They may also turn to alcohol or substance use as a coping method. This in turn may lead to sexual disinhibition and decreased ability to negotiate safer sex.

Peer Influences

Research has indicated that individuals are more likely to engage in safer sexual behaviors if they perceive support for risk reduction among their peers and community (Adib et al. 1991, Kelly et al. 1990). Perceived support may make it easier to initiate discussions about safer sex and negotiate safer sexual relations.

Substance Use

Many individuals use alcohol and other substances to cope with anxiety, depression, and other psychological distress. It is not unusual to hear about someone having a couple of drinks to "work up the courage" to approach an attractive potential partner. Although the alcohol and other substances may function to reduce anxiety, they can also reduce inhibitions, interfere with judgment, and increase the likelihood of risky sexual behaviors.

Factors for Women

Specific factors need to be considered when counseling women about safer sex. For example, mental health professionals need to remember that women inherently have less control over condom use than their male partners since they do not wear the condom. Risk reduction involves not only her decision to protect herself, but her ability to convince her partner to use a condom. Many women may be concerned that suggesting risk-reduction activities may indicate to her partner that he is not trusted or may result in his accusing her of promiscuity. In addition to these emotional aspects, the balance of power in a woman's relationship with a man impacts her ability to negotiate risk reduction. Women have reported factors such as economic dependence, safety concerns (for herself and her children), fears of rejection and loneliness, and survival concerns as inhibiting risk-reduction efforts (Rhodes et al. 1992).

THERAPIST ISSUES

As the AIDS epidemic continues, it becomes imperative that therapists learn to speak directly with their clients about sexual behaviors. Many mental health professionals receive little training on human sexuality or psychotherapeutic interventions targeting sexual behaviors. Consequently, many clinicians feel uncomfortable talking about sexual activities with their clients. Contributing to this reluctance may be a lack of knowledge about sexual behaviors, a lack of experience in openly discussing sex with clients, biases held toward the client, or the therapeutic style of the clinician.

When working with HIV seronegative and -positive clients, mental health professionals must examine their own beliefs and attitudes about the clients. Biases regarding HIV serostatus, sexual orientation, premarital sex, drug use, alternative sexual behaviors, and fears of contagion can impact a clinician's ability to work effectively. For example, the therapist who believes that an HIV-seropositive person should abstain from *all* sexual contact with others will be less effective in reducing the risks of a sexually active seropositive client than a clinician who believes that an HIV-positive person can negotiate and maintain safer sexual relations.

During training activities with mental health professionals, one issue that frequently arises is clinician biases regarding the sexual behaviors of clients. Clients may report sexual behaviors the clinician has not practiced or is unfamiliar with. The clinician thus may not understand the meaning of the activity for the individual and may discount the importance attached to that behavior. For example, a clinician who has little experience working with gay men may believe that giving up anal sex is a small sacrifice to protect oneself from HIV infection. As discussed earlier, anal sex may have many meanings for the client and may be as important to that client as vaginal intercourse is to a heterosexual client. Would that same therapist believe that giving up vaginal intercourse is a small sacrifice?

Integrating safer-sex training into psychotherapy may also be a challenge for the therapist based on his or her therapeutic style. For some clinicians a directive, active technique may not fit well with their usual approach in psychotherapy. Educational efforts during psychotherapy sessions may challenge the therapist's typical thoughts and beliefs about the role of the clinician, boundaries in the therapeutic relationship, and appropriate interventions. Adopting a "teaching style" during sessions may be difficult for some therapists. Some therapists choose to wait until the client brings up HIV-risk-related materials to address this in treatment. However, the therapist needs to examine whether this approach is actually colluding with the client to avoid the discussion and examination of HIV-risk behaviors or whether a client may interpret this approach as an endorsement to avoid these issues. For some therapists the challenge becomes one of integrating educational efforts into their work in a way that is comfortable for both parties in the therapeutic dyad.

INTEGRATING SAFER-SEX TRAINING INTO PSYCHOTHERAPY

Educating Yourself

To effectively educate clients, a therapist needs to educate him- or herself about HIV, safer sex, and related issues. In addition to reading this and other books, it is a good idea to attend HIV training workshops in your area, contact community-based AIDS service agencies for additional information, and consult with other professionals. By educating yourself, you will be able to provide your clients with accurate information and access to resources. For example, it is important not only to talk with some of your clients about using condoms but to provide information about their proper use. If discussing correct condom use is inappropriate during therapy sessions, written information, available from many HIV/AIDS community education programs, can be provided.

Taking a Sex/Drug-Use History

A sex and drug-use history is beneficial for the client and the therapist in several ways: it can serve as a mechanism to educate about HIV risks, determine current risk behaviors and risk-reduction efforts, provide information on the meaning of sex, and determine attitudes about changing behaviors to reduce risk. To determine the need for training in safer sex, the therapist needs to assess the client's sexual behaviors and drug use, current and past. Although taking a client's general history is an integral part of any clinician's training and work, a detailed sexual history may often be overlooked. A sexual history can easily be incorporated into a general pretreatment assessment. If a therapist uses a written questionnaire at the beginning of treatment, sexual history and safer-sex questions can easily be added to this procedure. The therapist can then follow up on the client's responses to clarify HIV risks and determine appropriate interventions. This method can be helpful in several ways:

1. Sexual behaviors are often uncomfortable to talk about directly. This method allows the client to respond initially in writing, which may be less threatening.
2. This sets the tone that sexual behaviors are important and can be discussed openly in sessions.
3. This procedure allows the therapist to determine the client's current knowledge about HIV and how he or she defines safer sex. The therapist should ask not just if the

client is protecting him- or herself, but how he or she is going about it.

4. The clinician can also begin to understand the client's thoughts and feelings about sex and risk reduction. Questions might include "What are your thoughts about safer sex?" "How did it feel to change your sexual behaviors?" "How successful have you been?"

Two factors are important in obtaining an accurate sex history. First, it is important to assess behaviors, not labels. The clinician who asks a male client if he is gay is assessing the man's sexual identity, not his behavior. There are many men who engage in sex with other men but do not self-identify as gay or identify with the gay community at large (Doll et al. 1992). It would be more appropriate for the therapist to ask, "Have you ever had sex with another man?"

Second, it is important to have an accepting, nonjudgmental approach to successfully assess sexual and drug-use behaviors. People frequently find it hard to talk directly about sexual activities and feelings. In addition, individuals from sexual minorities and substance abusers have frequently experienced judgmental reactions, blaming attitudes, and rejection by others. These clients may be acutely aware of subtle indications of judgmental attitudes and may react quickly by discounting the "advice" of the counselor. A nonjudgmental attitude will increase the likelihood that the client will be comfortable and provide accurate information.

Safer-Sex Training

Safer sexual behavior training can be effectively incorporated into psychotherapy through a variety of exercises encouraging exploration, skill development, and decision making by the client. When discussing safer-sex strategies and reviewing attempts at change, it is important not to blame individuals for relapses to unsafe behaviors. Relapses occur in most areas of behavior change (e.g., dieting, exercise, controlling substance use) and may be a normal part of the behavior change process. Key concepts central to the development of safer-sex strategies and sample exercises are provided below.

Assisting Clients in Defining Acceptable Risk Levels

One of the challenges of working with an individual who may be at risk for HIV infection is to facilitate the client's exploration and definition of his or her personal acceptable level of risk. This requires that the client understand the risks associated with various sexual behaviors and decide what behaviors she or he will be comfortable engaging in. One way to begin this process is to instruct the client to make a list of sexual behaviors, categorizing each behavior as safe, less safe, or unsafe. Review this list with the client and correct any misperceptions. Next, encourage the client to list behaviors he or she is or is not willing to engage in, along with a brief description of their motives. During this process clients may discover ambivalent or mixed feelings about certain behaviors. This provides an opportunity to explore the client's feelings and allows them to make an informed decision about these sexual behaviors. Clients may also identify alternative low-risk sexual behaviors not previously considered.

Skills Training

Many individuals need to learn specific skills to successfully reduce their risk for HIV infection. The most common example of skills training is instructions on the correct method of using a condom. Step-by-step instructions are important to reduce the risk of HIV transmission through condom breakage or other accidental exposure. If the therapist feels uncomfortable discussing this issue with the client, or believes it is inappropriate, then written instructions can be provided. It is recommended that individuals be directed to practice on their own prior to sexual contact with others.

Negotiating Safer Sex

Directly communicating with a partner about sexual activities and negotiating safer sex is often unfamiliar, uncomfortable, and difficult for clients. In order to protect oneself, an individual needs to learn effective methods for discussing risk reduction with partners prior to the initiation of sex and to develop strategies to resist pressures to participate in unsafe activities. The role of a therapist is to help the client explore perceived barriers to safer-sex negotiation and facilitate the discussion of alternatives for overcoming these barriers. Often it is helpful for clients to rehearse safer-sex negotiation strategies through role-play exercises with the therapist. This provides the client with a safe environment to practice and improve negotiation skills and allows the therapist to provide immediate feedback and recommend alternative strategies. The therapist may need to consider integrating assertiveness training into treatment for some individuals, especially women.

Eroticizing Safer Sex

One of the major complaints about safer sex as voiced by individuals is that it is not as fun as unsafe activities. D'Eramo and colleagues (1988) reported that interventions based on erotic, sexually explicit, safer-sex techniques were more effective in reducing risk behaviors than information-based interventions. This suggests that clients need to learn that safer sex is not boring, but can be exciting, stimulating, and enjoyable. Sometimes we need to be reminded that stimulating areas other than the genitals can be sensual and pleasurable. In fact, our biggest sex organ is the brain. As a therapist, you can assist your clients in exploring and eroticizing safer sexual activities and increase the likelihood that they will maintain safer sexual relations.

Nongenital-focused activities are one type of exercise that can be assigned as "homework" to begin eroticizing safer sex. These assignments are similar to the sensate focus exercises prescribed by sex therapists. A therapist might begin by asking the client to think about and practice ways he or she likes to touch or be touched in nongenital areas. As described earlier, if the client is uncomfortable discussing these activities directly, have him or her make a list. If the client has a partner, both can be directed to practice touching nongenital areas in ways that do not pose a risk for HIV infection. Clients should pay attention to what types of touch (e.g., firm versus light pressure) and what areas they most enjoy having touched or touching. By completing these exercises, the client can identify pleasurable, erotic, non-genital sources of pleasure. Some clients may discover that areas they never considered erotic are actually quite sensitive to touch. Safe or safer genital stimulation, such as mutual masturbation or anal-digital (finger) contact, can slowly be incorporated into these exercises.

Writing exercises can also assist clients in eroticizing safer sexual behaviors. For example, ask clients to list and describe different ways to integrate condoms into their sexual interactions in a fun, sexy way. After completing this assignment, have them practice, and revise as necessary, with a partner. A similar assignment can be used to incorporate sex toys or videos into low-risk sexual activities.

Some individuals find that talking can function as a stimulant for sexual arousal and enhance the enjoyment of safer sexual contact. Some people enjoy "talking dirty"—describing what one is doing and or wants to do; others enjoy erotic storytelling or reading erotic literature while touching. One indirect indication of this is the recent surge of advertisements for telephone sex services. Although I hesitate to recommend such services as a regular safe sex outlet due to economic factors, some clients find noncommercial phone sex with a known partner exciting and gratifying.

Examining Reactions to Behavior Change

Regardless of the therapist's method of educating and working with a client to reduce risk, the client's feelings about changing his or her behavior must be explored. Clients often experience a variety of feelings when incorporating safer sex into their lives, such as loss, sadness, frustration, and anger. How a client manages these feelings may impact the success of the risk-reduction techniques. Examining current sexual behaviors may prompt some clients to review past sexual relationships, which may bring up old feelings and issues that should be addressed in the therapeutic setting.

Bibliotherapy

Bibliotherapy can be an effective method of educating the client about HIV risks and encouraging risk-reduction efforts. Numerous books, available at many libraries and bookstores, provide such information. For example, *The New Joy of Gay Sex* (Silverstein and Picano 1992), an updated version of the original 1977 book, provides extensive, detailed information on various gay sexual behaviors and methods for risk reduction. In addition, many community-based organizations (e.g., Gay Men's Health Crisis, San Francisco AIDS Foundation, AIDS Project Los Angeles) have developed brochures and pamphlets targeting individuals at risk for HIV infection. These brochures, written in nontechnical, easy-to-understand language, are inexpensive and can be ordered to distribute to clients.

Providing Referrals

Participation in ongoing support groups and contact with community agencies can be instrumental in HIV risk-reduction efforts. Research indicates that the attitudes toward safer sex of friends, peers, and/or the community impacts the individual's likelihood of engaging in safer sexual practices as well as prevents relapse to unsafe sex (Adib et al. 1991, Kelly et al. 1990). Many community-based organizations offer either ongoing or short-term groups that provide social support for HIV risk reduction. Other community organizations, such as The STOP AIDS Project, offer single-session risk-reduction groups. These groups are an excellent resource for clinicians, particularly therapists who are uncomfortable talking with clients about sexual behaviors.

CONCLUSION

As mental health professionals, it is our responsibility to work with our clients to reduce self-destructive behaviors. In the 1990s, unprotected, unsafe sex may qualify as a potentially self-destructive behavior for many clients. By behaviorally reducing their sexual risks, clients can effectively protect themselves from HIV infection. All therapists need to develop the skills to assess HIV risks, provide education, and assist clients in developing and implementing alternative behaviors. The therapist may need to educate him- or herself, examine his or her biases about client populations, and determine how to integrate risk-reduction training strategies into his or her personal therapeutic style. By not addressing these issues, a therapist may be contributing to a dangerous situation with potentially terrible consequences.

REFERENCES

Adib S., Joseph, J., Ostrow, D., and James, S. (1991). Predictors of relapse in sexual practices among homosexual men. *AIDS Education & Prevention* 3:293–304

D'Eramo, J., Quadland, M., Shattls, W., et al. (1988). The *"800 men" project: a systematic evaluation of AIDS prevention programs demonstrating the efficacy of erotic, sexually explicit safer sex education on gay and bisexual men at risk for AIDS.* Abstract presented at the Fourth International Conference on AIDS, Stockholm, Sweden, June.

Doll, L., Peterson, L., White, C., and Johnson, E. (1992). Homosexually and nonhomosexually identified men who have sex with men: a behavioral comparison. *Journal of Sex Research* 29:1–14.

Hays, R., Kegeles, S., and Coates, T. (1990). High HIV risk-taking among young gay men. *AIDS* 4:901–907.

Kelly, J., Murphy, D., Sikkema, K., and Kalichman, S. (1993). Psychological interventions to prevent HIV infection are urgently needed. New priorities for behavioral research in the second decade of AIDS. *American Psychologist* 48:1023–1034.

Kelly, J., St. Lawrence, J., Brasfield, T., et al. (1990). Psychological factors that predict AIDS high risk versus AIDS precautionary behavior. *Journal of Consulting and Clinical Psychology* 58:117–120.

Levy, J. (1993). Pathogenesis of human immunodeficiency virus infection. *Microbiological Reviews* 57:183–289.

Lifson, A., O'Malley, P., Hessol, N., et al. (1990). HIV seroconversion in two homosexual men after receptive oral intercourse with ejaculation: implications for counseling concerning safe sexual practices. *American Journal of Public Health* 80:1509–1511.

Rhodes, F., Wolitski, R., and Thorton-Johnson, S. (1992). An experiential program to reduce AIDS risk among female sex

partners of injection drug users. *Health and Social Work*
17:261–272.
Silverstein, C., and Picano, F. (1992). *The New Joy of Gay Sex*. New
York: HarperCollins.
Zimmerman, R., and Olson, K. (1994). AIDS-related risk behavior and behavior change in a sexually active, heterosexual
sample: a test of three models of prevention. *AIDS Education
and Prevention* 6:189–204.

3

Cognitive-Behavioral Treatment Strategies for Emotionally Distressed Asymptomatic Seropositives

CATHERINE M. FLANAGAN

In the last ten years, the social context of AIDS has changed dramatically. The cause of AIDS is known, and this information has had the effect of decreasing feelings of "undifferentiated vulnerability" (Martin and Dean 1993). There is also a better understanding of why certain sections of the population are more likely to contract HIV and this has led to selective efforts to disseminate information to these groups. Despite these developments, however, the fatality rate for those infected with HIV has not changed; people who are diagnosed HIV positive face almost certain death (see Forstein 1984). AIDS also continues to be a stigmatized disease, and prejudice toward homosexuals continues at a high level in the United States (Dean et al. 1992). Furthermore, many gay men have experienced multiple losses of lovers and friends or have had first-degree exposure to the course of illness and eventual death of a significant other. Consequently, receiving, and living with, a diagnosis of seropositivity constitutes a major challenge to an individual's coping resources (Mansson 1992, Schaefer and Coleman 1992, Siegal and Krauss 1991).

PERSONAL RESILIENCE: COPING WITH LIFE-THREATENING ILLNESS

Surprisingly, most people with life-threatening illnesses do not become clinically depressed (Cella and Perry 1988); in fact, it seems that for some people facing their mortality provides an opportunity for self-examination and personal growth. Taylor (1986), for example, interviewed women with breast cancer; most of them had undergone surgery, and the prognoses ranged from very good to poor. Three main coping strategies were identified: searching for meaning in an effort to understand why; attempting to regain mastery over the illness and their lives, thereby maintaining a sense of self-efficacy; and, finally, trying to rebuild self-esteem, frequently through self-enhancing comparisons to others. Similarly, Cohen and Lazarus (1979) developed a cognitive theory of adaptation based on the different challenges and tasks that face the chronically ill and the coping strategies needed to deal effectively with these challenges. Overall, it seems that the average person's ability to assimilate and accommodate to profound change is striking. In this context the recent writings of the constructivist movement within cognitive psychology are worth noting, and in particular the accumulating information on self-organizing systems and how these dynamics play out in the arena of human change processes (see Mahoney 1993).

Given the extra challenges that people who are seropositive or who have AIDS have to face, it seems that the same holds true here also. In other words, most people who are HIV positive do not become depressed (Burack et al. 1993, Lyketsos et al. 1993); even long-term survivors of AIDS display an "extraordinary psychological resilience" (Rabkin et al. 1993). A study by Siegel and Krauss (1991) explored the adaptive strategies of a group of seropositive gay men. In addition to dealing with the distinct possibility of a curtailed life span—and with others' reactions to their stigmatizing illness—these gay men developed many strategies for maintaining physical and psychological well-being. What is striking about these self-initiated adaptations is not that the strategies were always effective, but they again seem to bear witness to the adaptive capabilities and resourcefulness of the average human being. It seems fair to suggest that, when under extreme pressure, people's normal coping mechanisms go into overdrive. For example, persons whose normal coping style is avoidant will automatically endeavor to cope through functional denial; people who cope through compensation will be seen to put extra effort into overtly coping and problem solving. In summary, under pressure, we do tend to contend with the stressful situations we encounter.

As a result of this natural adaptation to stressful life events, clinical distress or depression are not normal responses to having HIV infection (Perry and Fishman 1993) and therefore can be better conceptualized as treatable disorders. If clinical levels of depression and distress are not the expected response to life-threatening illness in general and those infected with HIV in particular, why then do some people fail to cope when under pressure? The answer seems to lie in the existence of maladaptive underlying schemas, or underlying vulnerabilities, which are triggered and highlighted in times of extreme pressure. When a person's normal coping mechanisms are not robust enough to click automatically into healthy overdrive, their underlying fragility is exposed. For example, a study by Perry and colleagues (1990) revealed that many individuals at perceived risk for AIDS may be vulnerable to depression. The lifetime rates for mood disorder in this population were roughly seven times higher than an age-matched community sample. Despite these rates, however, more than 70 percent of these subjects *did not* have current *DSM-III-R* Axis I psychopathology. Markowitz and colleagues (1992), in identifying useful aspects of short-term interpersonal therapy in the treatment of

HIV-positive patients, also acknowledged the existence of sub-chronic characterological disorders among their patients. In other words, in many cases there is an underlying core-level vulnerability that can be activated in extreme circumstances. If clinical levels of distress and depression are not the expected responses to being seropositive but are caused by preexisting vulnerabilities, then these latent vulnerabilities—erroneous beliefs and maladaptive schemas—can be identified and explored in therapy and patients can learn to cope in more effective ways.

DEPRESSION OR DISTRESS?

In my clinical experience working with seropositive patients, I have observed two main styles of dysfunctional coping; one leads to depression, the other to clinical levels of anxiety and distress. What determines the response are the individual's idiosyncratic underlying vulnerabilities (see Young 1990 for a more detailed discussion of schema-level vulnerability). Activation of core-level beliefs and maladaptive schemas leads to a systematic biasing of information processing. There can be a distortion of *external* information, such as communications and interactions with other people, and of *internal* information, such as bodily sensations and minor aches and pains. In cases of both depression and anxiety there is a perceived loss of control, but the dysfunctional coping styles and thought patterns of depressed and distressed clients are very different and consequently need to be addressed differently in therapy.

Distress

When people are highly anxious, all the normal, healthy, survival mechanisms go into overdrive. This can be self-defeating in that the responses that generally function to protect the person from threat become maladaptive when excessively or incorrectly activated.

The coding system in high anxiety involves a hypervigilance for, and selection of, data relevant to danger, an overinterpretation of danger, and increased access to danger themes in memory. Decisions are made quickly, and tend to be overinclusive in their discrimination of both threatening external stimuli (e.g., loud noises, bad weather) *and* internal physiological reactions (e.g., shortness of breath, palpitations). Anxious people tend to overestimate the risk and magnitude of perceived danger and cannot correct their misinterpretations using logic or evidence. Catastrophization is pervasive, and consequently things easily and quickly escalate. Highly anxious people also have difficulty recognizing cues of safety, or other evidence that could serve to decrease their perceived threat of danger. They also underestimate their own ability to cope. Instead, they feel scared, vulnerable, overwhelmed, and helpless—as if waiting for the other shoe to drop.

Depression

Depressed people also distort both their external and internal realities, but in a different way. There is an overpowering sense of defeat and loss. They perceive themselves as inadequate, deserted, or worthless. The world holds no pleasure. They feel helpless and the future seems hopeless. This decreased sense of control and self-efficacy leads to expectations of failure as well as to a perceived inability to cope with the consequences of these expected failures. Motivation is consequently eroded—what is known as "a paralysis of the will." Depressed people often see themselves as totally incompetent; consequently, the difficulty of everyday tasks is magnified out of proportion. Indecision and procrastination result from beliefs to the effect that they will make the wrong choice or that they cannot trust their own judgment. There is frequently self-loathing and self-blame. The physiological manifestations of depression are well known, among them diminished libido, fatigue, and inertia. There can be weight loss due to food restriction, or weight gain due to being more sedentary and/or eating in a nondiscriminating way. Depressed people frequently sleep a lot, or their sleep cycle can be very erratic. In anxiety things speed up; in depression everything grinds to a halt.

INTERVENTION STRATEGIES

When faced with illness and death, many explicit rules for living that derive from an individual's organization of reality are called into question. This can be confusing and frightening, and core-level beliefs are frequently triggered. As previously stated, whether people are depressed or clinically distressed, there is a common experience of loss of control. Thus the goal in both cases is to reestablish a sense of agency and self-efficacy. The first step in this process is to help them regain their objectivity. This is what is lost when the faulty coding system clicks into place, but is essential to be able to evaluate one's situation. The reality of being seropositive cannot be changed, but people can learn to cope more effectively with the challenges and changes their HIV status inevitably brings. This can make a huge difference in the quality of one's emotional and physical well-being.

Coping tools that are commonsense and practical are essential at such times. Short-term focused interventions such as cognitive therapy help people to make sense of the changes that are taking place in the different areas of their lives as well as in their perception of themselves. Cognitive therapy provides a plausible explanation for why they are depressed or anxious. It places a high value on time by focusing on here-and-now difficulties, thereby equipping people with cognitive and behavioral coping strategies to address the real challenges they are facing. My experience has been that clients quickly become engaged by the uncomplicated, problem-focused rationale of cognitive therapy and subsequently experience enough early symptom relief to maintain their motivation and commitment. As their sense of control and agency returns, helplessness and hopelessness diminish. Reempowerment and facilitation of perceived control are highly potent ingredients at this stage of therapy.

One of the most effective tools is the systematic use of Daily Records of Dysfunctional Thoughts. Negative automatic thought sequences and the feelings they trigger are systematically recorded by the patient. Repeated cognitive distortions are identified, and rational responses that provide a more objective and realistic perspective are generated. By tracking repeated thought sequences over a period of time and in a variety of problem situations, information concerning the subtle patterns and themes that constitute the individual's underlying vulnerabilities is gradually accumulated. When the severity of the depression or anxiety state has been reduced, the latent vulnerabilities are addressed. Erroneous core beliefs and maladaptive schemas are identified, explored, and challenged in session and by the client's testing out new ways of operating in the real world. Effecting changes at this level is more difficult to accomplish because of the natural resistance to letting go of familiar modus operandi—however self-defeating—but is essential in preventing future relapses into depression or distress. A number of clinical tools and strategies are used to facilitate this process; one is the *Vertical Arrow Technique* (Beck et al. 1979), discussed later in the chapter (see page 56). Patients gradually gain the ability to objectively evaluate the usefulness or validity of their own underlying beliefs and expectations, particularly those that drive the biased information processing systems in both depression and anxiety.

Problem-Focused and Emotion-Focused Coping

Because of the core-level nature of the issues these clients are dealing with, I have also found it helpful throughout the therapy process to repeatedly make the distinction between, as well as emphasize the importance of, problem-focused *and* emotion-focused coping (Lazarus and Folkoyan 1984). Problem-focused coping skills (i.e., defining situations as problems or challenges and generating solutions) are not enough to help people who are faced with a life-threatening illness to get in touch with and express the legitimate pain they are often experiencing. Our culture tends to trivialize distress (Lazarus 1985), and cognitive therapy itself has frequently been misconstrued as a therapy that deals primarily with the problem-focused aspects of coping. People need to know that it is not only okay but appropriate to feel scared or confused; that not all, or even most, negative feelings are the result of faulty cognitive processing; and that this is not a sign of weakness on their part, but of being human (see Mahoney 1991). Frequently people need to just let go of a flood of sadness or fear, or to vent feelings of pent-up frustration and anger—feelings they may have been holding in for fear of losing control, or of looking like a coward. In my sessions there have been many unexpected outpourings of sorrow and fear, of disappointment and bitterness; I have learned how essential it is to be flexible—to meet these people where they are at—at such times. To enforce structure, or to try to stick to a preplanned agenda, is not to legitimize their feelings or to validate what they are going through. (Again the growing constructivist literature suggests that a different, but equally important, kind of healing takes place at such times [see Mahoney 1993].)

   In summary, clients who are HIV positive can utilize the rational tools of standard cognitive therapy to help them differentiate between expectable levels of sadness and distress and the profound negative thinking of depression or the exaggerated hypervigilance of clinical anxiety. Equally important, however, they also frequently need a safe place where they can allow themselves to be vulnerable, where they can show how truly raw they feel inside, or how understandably scared or helpless they feel in the face of impending illness and death. Both experiences are necessary to help them regain their sense of control and deal with the real world in a more effective way, as well as to continue the process of emotional adaptation and reorganization of the self.

CLINICAL EXAMPLES

Two case studies are presented to help elucidate the previous discussion regarding distressed and depressed clients. I have chosen them to illustrate the common theme of perceived loss of control and how it can manifest differently (i.e., in either high levels of anxiety or in clinical depression). In both cases there was an underlying, preexisting vulnerability that was triggered in the face of dealing with the prospect of a life-threatening illness. Through these examples I hope to convey the diversity and complexity of their individual histories and coping styles. I also describe the gradual unfolding of the layers of thoughts, beliefs, and maladaptive schemas. Cognitive therapy provides clients with both a comprehensive conceptualization (i.e., an explanation of their personal distress) and the clinical tools to explore their idiosyncratic vulnerabilities, thereby regaining emotional equilibrium and a sense of control over their lives.

Case Example 1: Distress

John was a handsome, successful 30-year-old gay man who came into therapy because of high anxiety due to his HIV status and related feelings of vulnerability to illness. He had been diagnosed HIV positive two years before, but had become severely distressed only about a month before our first meeting, when his CD-4 count had reached 400—a figure he had previously defined as "the borderline." Since then, he had become hypervigilant to all physical sensations: any breathlessness, aches, or pains were seen as "symptoms." He was taking massive doses of vitamins, and wearing extra layers of clothes to protect himself from the cold and germs. He felt completely out of control, and terrified at the prospect of contracting a common cold or flu, then pneumonia, and of dying rapidly. In our first session John responded extremely enthusiastically to the cognitive model. He said he wanted to be my "star patient." As a consequence, his homework assignments (Daily Thought

Records) were excellent; he clearly captured the thought sequences fueling his distress. The following were his thoughts and feelings (based on a scale from 0 to 100) one morning when he woke feeling "slightly off-color":

Automatic Thought	Feeling
I'm really sick this time.	Overwhelmed 80
The virus must be active.	Frightened 80
All these aches and pains are definitely AIDS precursors.	Helpless 75
I will be sick and in the hospital soon.	Frightened 75
People are going to suspect something— I'm starting to look a little diseased.	Ashamed 60
I know this is the virus.	Scared 95
My health is getting worse.	Anxious 95
I'm under a lot of work stress—that will weaken my system even more.	Overwhelmed 60
I can't cope with all this.	Desperate 80
I wish I could just get sick and die— get it all over with.	Helpless 90
There is no hope that I will ever be cured.	Hopeless 80

John found the rational response technique* extremely helpful in generating some objectivity on his distress. For

---

*Rational Response Checklist:
1. What is the evidence?
2. What is another way of looking at this? (Cognitive reframe)
3. What's the best, worst, most likely outcome?
4. What can I do?

example, he wrote out the following rational responses to the negative thought sequence above.

Rational Response: I have no evidence that I am sick. I just feel a little off-color, which makes sense considering how hard I've been working. My body is telling me it's tired. That's all. At best I'll feel better by this afternoon. At worst I'll feel worse, in which case I'll get a good night's sleep and see how I feel tomorrow. Overall I need to make some changes in my schedule.

Automatic Thought: The virus must be active. (Frightened 80)

Rational Response: I have no evidence that the virus is active. The symptoms I'm experiencing are no different than any other time that I've been tired. At worst, this is the beginning of something serious, in which case I'll only make things worse by panicking. Calm down, and wait and see what happens.

Automatic Thought: People are going to suspect something— I'm starting to look a little diseased. (Ashamed 60)

Rational Response: I have no evidence that people are beginning to suspect. As a matter of fact, everyone is telling me how great I look—which is pretty amazing considering how hard I've been pushing myself. I look a little pale this morning because I'm tired and I've seen very little daylight in the last week. Again, what I need to do is to make some changes in my schedule.

Generating rational responses, which provided John with an alternative, objective perspective, helped alleviate his anxiety. He learned to identify repeated cognitive distortions such as Jumping to Conclusions, Mental Filter, and All-or-Nothing Thinking. In addition to witnessing firsthand how these tendencies to catastrophize made his anxiety spiral, he saw how this in turn resulted in a decreased ability to concentrate and an inability to reality-check. As our sessions progressed, John felt more at ease and more in control. He made a concerted effort to change his schedule so that he had more time to rest and relax. He kept ongoing Daily Thought Records, and enjoyed the process of spotting his "negative tapes" in different situations. "It's great. I caught myself doing it again and I switched on my other [rational response] tape instead. This really works."

As the Daily Thought Records accumulated and therapy progressed, subtle themes began to emerge, the most prevalent of which was a tendency to push himself to the limit and ultimately to be self-destructive. This emerged from a Daily Thought Record in which he deliberately went to a friend's house on an evening when all of the inhabitants had come down with an aggressive flu: he wanted to test out his vulnerability/invincibility. When we discussed this at our next session, the origins of this self-defeating modus operandi became more apparent. As a child John had experienced both rejection and humiliation for being "girlish"; he always felt different and, in some undefined way, defective and vulnerable. As a consequence, he craved attention. When he was 8 years old, in an attempt to draw attention to himself "in a big way," he had rubbed himself with poison ivy and was rushed to the local hospital. He had also gone through a period of setting fires, including his own home. As he grew older he compensated by pushing himself extremely hard at school; he had achieved very high grades and now had a thriving business. On a cognitive level his coping style was also compensatory: he had developed an elaborate fantasy world, to which he escaped at every possible opportunity. In one of his most elaborate fantasies he was incredibly wealthy and handsome and was desired by all the most desirable men in New York. This made him feel special, desirable, and inaccessible—and also allowed him to avoid the pain of his inner loneliness and insecurity. Both of these strategies (behavioral *and* cognitive) helped him to survive as a child and adolescent but at this time they were becoming self-defeating and were in fact adding to his distress. He was working extremely long hours, but actually derived very little personal satisfaction from his success. He was very handsome, but did not see himself as such. Finally, he had always avoided spending much time alone but recently was drawn to morbid negative fantasizing concerning his own death—vivid visual images of his last dramatic moments and of his own funeral, all of which resulted in stimulating feelings of panic.

A more self-destructive aspect of these maladaptive coping modes then emerged. When truly frightened, John either binged or had unsafe anonymous sex. His weight had always been inconsistent: he ate when he felt anxious and out of control and had gained 15 pounds since hearing of his "borderline" CD-4 count. He said that he had engaged in unsafe sex to prove his invincibility and to escape from the awful feelings of raw fear. "I just want to self-destruct. I just can't stand feeling so out of control." Afterwards, he always felt disgusted with himself and even more scared.

When we put all the pieces together, his self-destructive behavior started to make more sense to John. He found tracing the cycle of negative thoughts, feelings, and impulsive behavior, followed by feelings of self-disgust, extremely reassuring. Until then it had seemed like "all different pieces that didn't hang together but left me feeling even more out of control." We constructed a flash card, which he carried with him at all times; looking at it would interrupt the onset of the negative feelings and thoughts.

Flash Card: The flash card he used included the following messages: "Calm down. Gather your thoughts. You are in control. Having either unsafe sex or bingeing right now will only make you feel more out of control. Why make the situation worse when you can make it better? Anxiety is a normal response—self-destruction is not. The decision is yours. Just stay with it and it will pass."

For the first time in his life he felt truly in control. He gained a tremendous sense of self-esteem from protecting himself in this way. Therapy became a process of real self-healing as opposed to one of gaining my approval. When he felt overwhelmed, John gradually learned to stay with, and experience, his feelings of panic. If he was really "freaked," he called me. He also began to share his feeling with his friends and family, and to let himself be cared for by them. He had always acted as if he was invincible, but actually felt like a fraud because he was so empty and anxious inside. In our second-to-last session, he received the results of his most recent CD-4 count. It had dropped again by a few points. He was upset and cried at the beginning of our session. He felt scared and alone, but he was able to see that these feelings were understandable *and* that he was not alone. He was then able to muster his problem-solving skills to do his best to protect and take care of himself rather than to self-destruct.

Case Example 2: Depression

Mary was a 28-year-old Hispanic mother of two. She had discovered her HIV status three years previously when her newborn was diagnosed seropositive. It turned out that her husband-to-be, the father of her child, was bisexual and had infected her. She called off the wedding, quit her job, and plummeted into a deep depression, which included a suicide attempt. That was eighteen months before; she was now severely depressed again. Her CD-4 count was 278. When I first met Mary she appeared to be in a state of shock: "I feel unreal." "I don't want this to be happening to me." "I want to get out of my body." "I feel so ashamed to have this." She felt she could not trust anyone. She told me that she had been such a positive person, that nothing could ever get her down. Now she just did not care. She spent her days sitting in front of the TV, giving her little boy the minimum amount of care and attention.

When I explained the rationale of the cognitive approach, she latched onto it with a desperate enthusiasm. Her Daily Thought Records revealed the true extent of her pain, which she so much wanted to cast off and to feel like herself again.

Automatic Thought	Feeling
I would have been married already and started a new life.	Terrible 90
We had so many friends together, as a starting couple.	Sad 60
All the good things—I thought everything was going to fall into place at last.	Devastated 100
He threw it all away—he messed up both our lives.	Hate 90
I wonder, I hope, he is going through what I am.	Angry 80
He didn't care enough to protect himself or me.	Angry 85
We're all involved now—I am and the baby too.	Empty 90
He destroyed it all.	Sad 100

In her first few weeks in therapy there was a visible change. Mary put her heart and soul into feeling better. By keeping a Daily Activity Schedule, she began to reidentify the things that she was good at, for example, home improvements; she also gained some pleasure from her appearance and meeting friends. She dressed up for our sessions. She started to contact friends again. She found that keeping Daily Thought Records and generating rational responses were enormously helpful in giving her an alternative perspective on her situation, which consequently enabled her to shift her mood. Mary found it especially important to focus on the present and future rather than going over the past. She enjoyed the process of identifying cognitive distortions such as *Labeling* ("I am a dirty person") and *Personalizing* ("It's my fault—I should have seen through him"). I felt uncomfortable with how quickly she was improving, but endeavors on my part to pinpoint her underlying vulnerability to depression were met with resistance. She insisted it came "out of the blue," so I waited and watched as she consolidated her gains. Using the Vertical Arrow Technique to explore underlying beliefs revealed many rules to do with life's fairness and unfairness: people *should* treat other people with respect and caring, everybody *should* try to be in good humor all the time and put the best face forward, she *should* not make mistakes. When we explored this tendency to blame herself for her HIV status, the following sequence was revealed using the Vertical Arrow Technique (Beck et al. 1979):

Vertical Arrow Technique

"It's my fault—I *should* have seen through him."

"And if that were true, what would it mean to you? Why would it upset you?"

"That would mean that I deserve what I got because I wanted so much to be happy that I didn't see him for what he was."

"And if that were true. . . ?"

"I *should* have asked more questions, rather than thinking he was a good guy."

"And if that were true. . . ?"

"Even if I had asked, he would not necessarily have told me the truth. He *should not* have pretended that he was something he wasn't."

"And if that were true. . . ?"

"Because people *shouldn't* lie to other people or deceive them."

"And if that were true. . . ?"

"People should treat other people with respect—otherwise there's no point. You just can't trust anyone anymore."

"And if that were true. . . ?"

"That would mean that I'd have to stay completely alone forever to be safe."

"And if that were true. . . ?"

"That would be awful. It would just not be fair. I hate to be alone. I get so down when I am alone. I shouldn't have to be alone."

> Initially, Mary was not open to hearing any feedback to the effect that many of her beliefs put enormous pressure on her to be in good humor all the time as well as set her up for disappointment when others did not fulfill her expectations. She said that she didn't really mean that she avoided being alone, that she just preferred company.
>
> In our eleventh session Mary came in visibly distraught and said that "everything is falling apart." The father of her child was threatening to gain custody by lying about her competence as a mother and about her emotional stability. She felt that she could not trust anyone, that there was nobody there to protect her. She said that she had not been

able to be open and honest with me because we would be meeting for only a limited period and it was so hard for her to trust anyone. Then she disclosed, for the first time in her life, repeated sexual abuse by her two brothers over many years, until, at the age of 16, she had married a man she did not love to get out of her home. The brothers had threatened that they would kill her if she told anyone. She did not trust her father either because he had cheated on her mother so she was afraid to tell him. She did not want to bring her mother any more sadness or disappointment. Her husband, in turn, was physically abusive; she left him three years later with her first child who was then 2 years old. It was seven years before Mary again trusted anyone enough to become involved in a relationship. She had then dated the father of her child for three years before deciding to commit to him; they had planned to marry after the birth of her baby. When she was told of her HIV status, the bottom fell out of her world. She had nothing left to fight for, or fight with. It all felt so unfair; there was nothing she could do this time to escape. She just sobbed and sobbed. She blamed herself for having been so naive, for having gone from one bad situation to another all her life. She blamed her parents for not having protected her and her partners for having taken advantage of her. She intermittently apologized to me for crying so much. I reassured her, put my arm around her, and told her that being able to get in touch with her feeling of sadness and despair was just as important in helping her to come to terms with all of this as being able to stand back and be objective and problem-focused. Cognitively and emotionally, Mary had developed an avoidant style to escape her inner pain. By compensating behaviorally (i.e., by keeping herself on the go all the time), she never allowed herself time to stop and think or feel. Now this long-term survival strategy was no longer working for her. She was raw and vulnerable and needed a safe place to deal with these awful feelings and be able to regroup and go on. I explained to Mary how we all develop survival strategies at an early age that actually do help us to cope with adversity but frequently get us stuck in repeated patterns and negative cycles at a later stage. I told her that she was wonderful to have survived such abuse and deprivation of protection, and that what had happened was not her fault. I also reassured her that her survival strategies— especially her resourcefulness and her ability to be positive and constructive—would serve her well in the future. This was all very comforting to her.

In our remaining sessions, in addition to being able to reharness her vital day-to-day coping abilities, Mary adopted a more realistic outlook. She continued to keep her Daily Thought Records, and was more open to the idea that her expectations of herself and of others had often been unrealistic. This saved her from many further minor disappointments. She also began the slower process of accepting her current situation and coming to terms with all that had happened to bring her to this point. She learned to be more discriminating about those in whom she placed her trust, which gave her a more real sense of control than she had experienced before. She became better at focusing on the present and future, and on living in the moment rather than in the past. She said that she felt more in touch with herself, and consequently did not feel the need to push herself quite so hard to always be in good humor and to keep on the go, to always look happy and be on top of things. She found a place for herself somewhere between the depths of depression that she had feared and avoided all her life, and the overly "Pollyanna" coping strategy that had helped her to avoid her inner pain but had actually prevented her from learning how to truly protect herself in the real world.

CONCLUSION

Most people with life-threatening illnesses, including those infected with the HIV virus, do not experience clinical levels of distress or depression. In general, people seem to have or develop ways of coping with both the emotional and practical aspects of their diagnosis or illness. These coping mechanisms are not always completely effective, but by and large can be viewed as healthy efforts to adapt to the demands of the situation. They reflect the individual's familiar coping style and the strategies the person has developed in the course of dealing with life's ups and downs. Most people continue to modify these coping mechanisms as they successfully make life transitions. When pressures and challenges are intense, these coping strategies are mobilized, and are visible in the individual's behavior and reactions. In other words, coping mechanisms become more intense and exaggerated when put to the test. People whose coping strategies are already fragile, and whose underlying schemas are maladaptive, sometimes simply cannot cope in extreme circumstances. These are the minority who become clinically distressed or depressed when they feel they are no longer in control of their lives. Consequently, the tools of standard cognitive therapy are highly appropriate and effective in giving them back a sense of objectivity and enabling them to regain a sense of agency and self-efficacy. Because of the core level of challenge that people with life-threatening illness have to face, they also have to be able to deal with intense, core-level emotional reorganization. For many, dealing with life and death issues—facing one's mortality—surprisingly creates a unique and positive opportunity for change and personal growth; ironically, for people with core-level vulnerabilities, this may be even more the case. Extreme adversity can provide an opportunity to truly reorganize or redefine the self, as in the case examples described, thereby allowing the person—and vulnerable individuals in particular—to function more adaptively and with a greater degree of openness to change than they had ever before, or might even otherwise have, experienced.

REFERENCES

Beck, A. T., Rush, J. A., Shaw, B. F., and Emery, G. (1979). *Cognitive Treatment of Depression*, p. 250. New York: Guilford.

Burack, J. H., Barrett, D. C., Stall, R. D., et al. (1993). Depressive symptoms and CD-4 lymphocyte decline among HIV-infected men. *Journal of the American Medical Association*, vol. 270, No. 21:2568–2573.

Cella, D. F., and Perry, S. W. (1988). Depression and physical illness. In *Phenomenology of Depressive Illness*, ed. J. J. Mann, pp. 33–51. New York: Human Services Press.

Cohen, F., and Lazarus, R. S. (1979). Coping with the stresses of illness. In *Health Psychiatry Handbook*, ed. G. C. Stone, F. Cohen, N. E. Adler, et al., pp. 217–254. San Francisco: Jossey-Bass.

Dean, L., Wu, S., and Martin, J. L. (1992). Trends in violence and discrimination against gay men in New York City, 1984–1990. In *Hate Crimes: Confronting Violence against Lesbians and Gay Men*, ed. G. Herek and K. T. Berrell, pp. 46–64. Newbury Park, CA: Sage.

Forstein, M. (1984). The psychosocial impact of the acquired immune deficiency syndrome. *Seminars in Oncology* 11:77–82.

Lazarus, R. S. (1985). The trivialization of distress. In *Preventing Health Risk Behavior in Promoting Coping with Illness*, ed. J. C. Rosen and L. J. Solomon, vol. 8, pp. 279–298. Vermont Conference on the Primary Prevention of Psychopathology. Hanover, NH: University Press of New England.

Lazarus R. S., and Folkoyan, S. (1984). *Stress, Appraisal and Coping*. New York: Springer.

Lyketsos, C. G., Hoover, D. R., and Giuccione, M. (1993). Depressive symptoms as predictors of medical outcomes in HIV infection. *Journal of the American Medical Association*, vol. 270, No. 21:2563–2567.

Mahoney, M. J. (1991). *Human Change Processes*. New York: Basic Books.

———— (1993). Theoretical development in the cognitive psychotherapies. *Journal of Counseling and Clinical Psychotherapy*, vol. 61, No. 2, 187–193.

Mansson, S. (1992). Dead-end or turning point: on homosexuality and coping with HIV. *Journal of Psychology and Human Sexuality*, vol. 5, 12:157–176.

Markowitz, J., Klerman, G., and Perry, S. W. (1992). Interpersonal psychotherapy of depressed HIV-positive outpatients. *Hospital and Community Psychiatry*, vol. 43, No. 9: 885–890.

Martin, J., and Dean, L. (1993). Effects of AIDS-related bereavement and HIV-related illness on psychological distress among gay men. A seven-year longitudinal study, 1985–1991. *Journal of Consulting and Clinical Psychology* 61:94–103.

Perry, S. W., and Fishman, B. (1993). Depression and HIV: how does one affect the other? *Journal of the American Medical Association*, vol. 270, No. 21:2609–2610.

Perry, S. W., Jacobsberg, L., and Fishman, B. (1990). Psychiatric diagnosis before serological testing for human immunodeficiency virus. *American Journal of Psychiatry* 147, 1:89–93.

Rabkin, J. G., Remien, R. H., Katofoff, L., et al. (1993). Resilience in adversity among long-term survivors of AIDS. *Hospital and Community Psychiatry*, vol. 44: No. 2, 162–167.

Schaefer, S., and Coleman, E. (1992). Shifts in meaning, purpose and values following a diagnosis of human immunodeficiency virus (HIV) infection among gay men. *Journal of Psychology and Human Sexuality*, vol. 5 (1–2):13–29.

Siegel, K., and Krauss, B. (1991). Living with HIV infection: adaptive tasks of seropositive gay men. *Journal of Health and Social Behavior*, vol. 32 (March) 17–32.

Taylor, S. E. (1986). *Health Psychology*. New York: Random House.

Young, J. E. (1990). *Cognitive Therapy for Personality Disorders: A Schema-Focused Approach*. Sarasota, FL: Professional Resources Exchange, Inc.

4

Psychotherapy with Dying Aids Patients and Their Significant Others

VICKI GLUHOSKI

Facing the inevitability of death is a challenge we all will confront. Extensive literature exists on this issue, but limited work has examined how to treat this challenge clinically in any population. Even fewer writings have specifically addressed psychotherapy for those dying of AIDS. This chapter has several goals: to delineate the prominent issues for those dying of AIDS, to outline treatment based on these needs, and to describe the challenges and interventions for the loved ones of AIDS patients. Particular issues that are addressed include finding meaning, spiritual needs, coping with physical discomfort, and managing interpersonal relationships.

A discussion of coping with dying would be remiss if the work of Elizabeth Kubler-Ross was deleted (see Rainey 1988 for a review, Wong et al. 1994). This frequently cited model, which has been subject to recent criticism, argues that the dying process consists of five stages and that all individuals proceed through these stages in a fixed sequence. In this model the first stage of denial and isolation is marked by a numbing and nonacceptance of impending demise. The second stage, anger, is characterized by rage at the unfairness of the situation and the search to understand why this is happening. Bargaining is the next stage, in which the individual seeks to reverse his or her fate by making promises and attempting to change. These avowals may be made to oneself, loved ones, medical staff, or God. As the person comes to recognize that he or she cannot change the inevitability of death, depression becomes prominent. In this stage the individual can no longer deny the changes taking place, including altered health status, diminished autonomy, and relinquished roles. The final stage in this model is acceptance. The individual eventually recognizes that he or she will soon die and accepts this fate peacefully.

Kubler-Ross's stage model is popular, but it has been critically reviewed and rejected. Schultz and Aderman (1974) argue that the model is too vague and rigid and that dying does not consist of a fixed system of responses. They are dissatisfied that measurements have not been developed to assess the stages and they also emphasize that the model was not based on rigorous research, but on a subjective interpretation. Corr (1993) also finds the stage model to be inadequate. He believes that it disregards individuality by rigidly prescribing what the person should experience. The model neglects preexisting attributes of the patient, ignores the unique features of their situation, and does not address their resources. Finally and most significantly, the model has never been validated empirically.

Rainey (1988) proposes that the dying process can be broken down into three phases: learning of the illness; "chronic living," which consists of the time from prognosis to the end stage; and finally the terminal phase, when the patient is close to death. Rainey does not suggest that certain tasks must be accomplished during these phases. Instead he offers this time-line as a general guide to demarcate significant transitions. This view might be more useful because it does not dictate what the patient must experience.

Although stage models have inadequately described emotional responses of the dying, some researchers have examined factors associated with distress in the terminally ill. In a sample of twenty dying patients, Smith and colleagues (1983) found that, overall, these patients reported a low-level fear of death. Age was significantly associated with fear in that as age increased, fear diminished, regardless of life expectancy. These researchers also examined depressive symptoms and found that none of the sample met criteria for clinical depression. Religiosity was also studied. It was found that strength or certainty of one's beliefs about an afterlife were more significant than the content of the belief. Patients who held strong beliefs about what happens after death, either positive or negative, were less fearful than subjects who were uncertain.

These findings have been replicated by others. Feifel and Branscomb (1981) also found that older and more religious patients held fewer fears of death. Nearness to death was again not significantly related to fear. Carey (1974) found that quality of spiritual beliefs was critical, similar to Smith and colleagues' (1983) construct of certainty of afterlife beliefs. Carey (1974; see also Gibbs and Achterberg-Lawlis 1978) also examined the importance of previous experience with a dying person. Patients who discussed death with a loved one who subsequently died, but were accepting of it, reported better adjustment with their own imminent death. Conversely, patients who lost a loved one who had been bitter about dying showed more distress about their own health decline.

Only one study has examined death anxiety in an HIV-positive sample. In a sample of ninety-four HIV-positive gay men (thirty-four asymptomatic, thirty-six with AIDS-related complex, and twenty-four with AIDS), Hintze and colleagues (1994) found that attitudes toward death were related significantly to state and trait measures of anxiety, and secondarily to a measure of depression. Variables that most strongly predicted death anxiety included state anxiety, depression, and having one's family aware of the diagnosis. Physical health status did not show a powerful relationship to death attitudes. Evidence also shows that receiving a diagnosis of HIV does not cause clinical depression, although feelings of sadness, anxiety, and fear often accompany the news. Markowitz and colleagues (1994) report that episodes of depression in HIV-positive gay men do not differ from HIV-negative gay men or the general population. In addition, the majority of men in their sample who were HIV-positive and depressed had a history of depression prior to HIV diagnosis.

These findings all suggest that facing one's own death is not universally associated with a defining set of emotional reactions. Although there is clear individual variability in response to the dying process, common themes and issues are also apparent. How people respond to these challenges may differ, but several shared aspects of the process may be seen across individuals. These themes include finding meaning, physical changes, and interpersonal relationships. A discussion of each of these issues and their treatment implications follows.

ISSUES ASSOCIATED WITH DYING

Finding Meaning and Existential Concerns

Taylor (1983) has suggested that adaptation to personally threatening life events includes three processes: seeking meaning, making efforts to gain control over the event in one's life, and attempting to restore one's self-view. She views the need to find meaning as an attempt at mastery. If the individual can understand and explain why the event occurred, it may lead to an enhanced sense of control and diminished vulnerability. More specifically, she argues that searching for meaning may produce a shifting of priorities and an altered belief system. For example, her work with breast cancer patients has shown that those who found positive meaning in the illness had less psychological distress.

Others have addressed the specific fears of the dying that may be the catalyst for the search for meaning. Weisman and Worden (1976) describe an "existential plight" that occurs with a diagnosis of a fatal disease (p. 1). They suggest that learning of the diagnosis leads to ruminating about life and death, raises questions about diverse life areas, and produces a new perspective on one's place in the world. They found that younger patients had more existential distress. These patients focused more on destroyed life plans and having to develop a different view of themselves, their relationships, and work goals (see also Tomer 1994; Wong et al. 1994). Rainey (1988) suggests that this transition may be less difficult if the person can maintain what had previously been meaningful, as well as retain significant aspects of identity before the illness.

In addition to focusing on what will be relinquished, the dying must also confront their beliefs about death and afterlife. Wong and colleagues (1994) suggest that death can be viewed as either a destruction of existence or a passage to another, better place. Those who hold the former view may be focused on conducting a purposeful life; those with the latter view may be somewhat less distressed about their own death. Morgan (1988) argues that all individuals hold a death system, or orientation to death. This system includes one's attitudes toward living and dying, concepts of death and afterlife, and beliefs about funerals and mourning rituals. This system has cognitive, emotional, and behavioral components. He believes that it is developed by both tangible experiences and philosophical stance. Although we all hold a death system, it most likely does not come to the forefront or may not be well formulated until we are faced with our own mortality.

Some work has begun specifically to examine meaning and existential concerns of people living with AIDS. Moynihan and colleagues (1988; see also Stulberg and Buckingham 1988) suggest that three factors are especially relevant: the youth of the patient, course of the disease, and the social context. Developmental norms of adults (25-50 years of age) living with AIDS typically include choosing/managing a career, developing long-term relationships, and forming an identity of oneself as an independent adult. For those who are dying, these opportunities may not be available. The young age of these patients may also mean that they have limited experience with loss and may be ill-prepared to confront these issues (Murphy and Perry 1988). Tross and Hirsch (1988) suggest that self-view may be altered because of changes in appearance and declining physical functioning. This may be associated with an enhanced sense of vulnerability and distress. The dying process contradicts the assumptions of youth: a long, healthy life, future goals, physical attractiveness, and autonomy. This process forces the individual to recognize that these expectations and goals may not be obtained.

The social environment of AIDS is different from other terminal illnesses and this may have an impact on existential concerns (Moynihan et al. 1988). The individual may face rejection, discrimination, or blame. He or she may have seen others die of AIDS and may be fearful of a similar painful death. Under such circumstances it may be difficult to maintain hope or deny how the disease progresses. In addition, some AIDS patients may feel guilty or blame themselves for contracting the illness. They may have become alienated from spiritual or religious outlets and may not be able to find comfort from these resources.

A significant aspect of this process is defining one's spiritual beliefs. A distinction may be made between religious and spiritual issues. Spirituality is defined by Speck (1989) as part of the search to answer and understand why events occur and to help find meaning. Resolving these questions may occur outside a religious context. However, religion may be the source for resolving these issues for some individuals. Religious practices may represent a tangible expression of one's spiritual philosophy.

Another critical opportunity to finding meaning in dying may occur through a life review. Erikson (see Tomer 1994 for a review) theorized that the final developmental task is reviewing one's life to determine whether it has been meaningful and fulfilling. A sense of integrity occurs if the individual believes that he or she led a satisfying life. Despair results if the individual has many regrets. The individual may be able to construe his or her experience in a framework so that integrity, a sense of peace, and meaningfulness can be obtained.

It is clear that resolving existential questions and finding meaning or understanding is a critical issue for the dying. The impact of not resolving these questions has never been studied and is worthy of future examination. Certain strategies to facilitate finding meaning are discussed later in this chapter. The possibility that patients might not be fully able to resolve their existential concerns is also addressed.

Physical Health Issues

In addition to existential concerns and shattered possibilities, the dying are faced with physical changes and discomfort. Fishman (1992) has outlined specific health issues of dying patients and has categorized them as either medical or personal/social threats. He defines medical threats as uncontrollable pain, narcotic addiction, mutilating surgery, treatment failure, physical disability, advancing disease, and approaching death. He views personal and social threats as a series of losses, including dignity, self-control, mental ability, social status, employment, financial resources, and independence.

Corr (1993) has discussed the needs of dying patients such as symptom relief, the stability of a supportive helping environment, ongoing medical attention, and the recognition that they will not be deserted. Corr advises that caregivers must be attentive to the patient and help him or her to define specific needs and how best to meet them. Others (Kelly and St. Lawrence 1988) have addressed some unique needs of AIDS patients, including access to sophisticated medical care, the opportunity to be a part of clinical research investigating new treatments, assistance with caretaking, housing, and legal and financial support.

Physical changes, such as Kaposi's sarcoma, ataxia, and diminished cognitive capacity, are symptoms of AIDS that challenge many patients living with the disease (Moynihan et al. 1988). These visible changes are tangible proof that one's health is deteriorating and this inevitability can no longer be denied. Such physical evidence may also cause the patient to be stigmatized or avoided by others. These symptoms signify a loss of attractiveness and desirability.

Pain and its management are also critical issues that must be addressed. Fishman (1992) suggests that the uncertainty of pain control can cause anxiety while the debilitating effects of pain diminish self-worth and lead to depression. In addition, anger may be experienced if the individual believes that his or her goals are blocked due to their pain. Naysmith and O'Neill (1989) believe that patients may interpret their pain as evidence that they are deteriorating and this realization can lead to the development of feelings of hopelessness and depression. They stress that diverse techniques are available for pain management, which may ease patients' distress. However, they acknowledge that it is more difficult to control other symptoms, such as appetite disturbance, vomiting, breathlessness, and general weakness.

Physical deterioration and pain sensations are ongoing issues that are relieved only by death. The chronicity and discomfort caused by these events may be frustrating, demoralizing, and lead to diminished affect. While the reality of these changes should not be denied or minimized, psychotherapy can be employed to alleviate some of the distress. These strategies are addressed later in this chapter.

Interpersonal Issues

The final realm to be discussed encompasses interpersonal relationships. Assisting a dying loved one may entail significantly altering roles (Naysmith and O'Neill 1989). A partner or parent may have to become a caregiver. Relationships that were previously based on an equal distribution of power and responsibility may become sharply skewed. In addition, relationships that were problematic in the past may become even more difficult with the additional stressors associated with the illness (Stulberg and Buckingham 1988). Long-term conflicts may resurface or be intensified. These prior difficulties may become a focus of treatment for the patient living with AIDS who wants to resolve or reconcile these conflicts.

Even if the patient has positive relationships with his or her loved ones, other problems may arise. The family may not recognize the extent of the patient's limitations and may make unrealistic demands or offer inadequate assistance. Conversely, they may be too protective and involved and thus diminish the patient's sense of autonomy and competence. With sexual partners, an altered means of obtaining intimacy and sexual satisfaction becomes necessary. The patient cannot provide all that he or she had previously given. A shifting of roles occurs and neither partner may have his or her needs satisfied (see Moynihan et al. 1988).

The patient may also have the task of planning for a secure future for his or her family. Activities such as writing a will or arranging benefits for a partner or children force the patient to acknowledge the severity and finality of his or her condition (see Moynihan et al. 1988). These tasks may also ease the patient's anxieties somewhat if he or she can ensure that the loved ones will have a secure future. A sense of competence or accomplishment may result if the patient can see how he or she has provided for and helped others.

Family members have different issues in caring for a dying

loved one, which will be discussed at length later in this chapter. In the preceding pages a number of issues have been raised about the needs and challenges associated with the dying process. Several questions are addressed in the following section: How should therapy be structured with a patient dying of AIDS? How can a sense of control and meaning be achieved? Finally, how can fear and pain be handled?

PSYCHOTHERAPY FOR THE DYING

General Themes and Process

A focused and goal-directed approach may be most useful with the dying patient (Lomax and Sandler 1988). This strategy will help to alleviate distress most directly and immediately and enhance a patient's sense of control. Several authors have suggested appropriate treatment goals that address physical, social, spiritual, and psychological needs. For example, Corr (1991) believes that treatment should facilitate the following: minimization of physical pain, enhancement of autonomy, maintenance of relationships, and development of a spiritual philosophy. Morgan (1988) concurs with Corr but also underscores that patients should have the opportunity to satisfy last wishes. This process may involve defining new goals or recognizing what previous desires have gone unfulfilled and how to complete them (Lomax and Sandler 1988).

Sherr (1989a) has adapted the general literature on the tasks of dying to AIDS patients and argues that treatment must include three components: (1) a life review in which the patient tries to examine the positive aspects of his or her life; (2) reconciliation of practical issues such as caretaking and finances; and (3) instruction in problem-solving skills so that acceptable solutions are likely to be identified, thus helping the patient be an active coper.

Although the therapist should retain a positive and hopeful stance, he or she must acknowledge the patient's realistic fears and concerns. The therapist should not deny the poor prognosis as this does not serve the patient's best interests and would be invalidating (Kelly and St. Lawrence 1988). Despite the severity of the patient's condition, the teaching of coping strategies can diminish the patient's distress.

An initial assessment is necessary to determine whether the patient is appropriate for psychotherapy. Some patients may have their needs adequately met through religious or philosophical associations and can be referred to those sources. Others may not have the cognitive capacity necessary if intervention is begun too late in the disease process. Finally, the therapist should examine the timing of psychotherapy: if treatment starts long before death, the therapist may become an additional significant other from whom separation is difficult. However, treatment should begin early enough in the disease process for the therapist to develop a thorough conceptualization of the individual, rather than just identifying the patient as a person with AIDS without attending to his or her unique attributes (Feigenberg 1975).

It is important to allow the patient to set the pace of the psychotherapy (Sherr 1989b). Initially the patient may deny or avoid discussing his or her impending death (Moynihan et al. 1988). Denying certain aspects of one's condition may be adaptive at times when the threat may appear overwhelming (Rainey 1988). The therapist must be attuned to when the patient is using denial as a strategy to titrate overwhelming emotions and when it reflects a complete avoidance of realistic threats. The former may represent a useful coping technique that should not be taken away from the patient, while the latter may be maladaptive.

Therapists working with dying patients must be flexible, as standard therapy expectations may not be applicable (Feigenberg 1975). For example, as the patient deteriorates, a fifty-minute session will most likely be too long; its length may be determined by the patient's energy level. The therapist may also have to act as a liaison, and have more contact with medical staff and family than is typical in individual therapy. In addition, because of the unpredictable course of AIDS and unexpected additional stressors, the therapist must be prepared to work with a host of changing emotions. For example, a patient may become anxious when a new symptom develops, sad when he learns a friend has died of AIDS, or overwhelmed with insurance paperwork. The therapist cannot set rigid therapeutic agendas or goals. The ever-changing environment and needs of the patient must be incorporated into the therapy process.

Finally, the therapist's own reactions to working with this population must be noted (McKusick 1988). Psychotherapy with patients dying from AIDS can be meaningful and rewarding but it can also cause sadness, demoralization, and helplessness. Acknowledging these reactions, both to oneself and the patient, may aid in the therapeutic process. As the therapist becomes aware of his or her reactions, he or she can monitor them and ensure they do not have a deleterious effect on the work. By sharing some of one's own sadness about losing the relationship with the patient, the therapist is demonstrating coping behavior as well as expressing that the client has had a positive impact on the therapist. This may serve to heighten the alliance as well as provide a model of coping.

Enhancing Personal Control and Meaning

Taylor (1983) has suggested that having some control over one's care is critical for dying patients because it contributes to a sense of mastery. In addition, a sense of control might aid in diminishing perceived helplessness that may be associated with anxiety or depression (Kelly and Murphy 1992). Enhancing the patient's control can be achieved through several strategies. Of primary importance is helping the patient to identify where he or she has choices and different options. For example, the patient can be involved in decisions about pain medication, various medical procedures, and whether or not to sustain life at a certain point (Moynihan et al. 1988). This active participation in planning may challenge the patient's view of him- or herself as passive and without any decision-making authority. A mechanism to enhance this sense of involvement is information seeking (Taylor 1983). The patient who learns about different terminologies and options can be involved more completely in treatment decisions. Subsequently, the disease may seem less vague and confusing, which may lessen anxiety.

Teaching active problem-solving skills can also enhance a sense of control. As the patient learns how to generate, evaluate, and implement solutions, a sense of helplessness may be avoided or alleviated. Cognitive therapy techniques may also be used to evaluate how the patient may be distorting or underestimating how much control he or she actually has over medical care and disease progression. In addition, the patient can be taught how to use these techniques during times of negative thinking. Recognizing that affect can easily be enhanced by the patient may also contribute to his or her sense of mastery.

Prior coping style must be assessed. Although the stressor is different, it is likely that the patient will try to cope with strategies that have worked before (Rainey 1988). Such techniques may be well learned and the preferred choice. Conversely, if the patient has coped poorly with previous stressors, new or varied techniques may have to be taught. As the patient's needs change, diverse strategies may have to be implemented (Kelly and Murphy 1992). Initially the patient may prefer to deny the severity of his or her condition, but this avoidance may become problematic or difficult to maintain. He or she may have to learn techniques for recognizing the deterioration in health without becoming overwhelmed.

Some empirical work has examined coping strategies of terminally ill patients. Weisman and Worden (1976) looked at the association between coping style and psychological distress in recently diagnosed cancer patients. They found that lower distress was related to seeking information, discussing one's fears, and reframing negative aspects. Passivity, pessimism, and not discussing concerns were associated with poorer outcome.

Similar results were obtained by Feifel and colleagues (1987). They examined differences in coping between patients with life-threatening illnesses (cancer or heart disease) or nonlife-threatening diseases (arthritis or dermatitis). They found that more seriously ill patients utilized more active strategies, including information seeking, redefining the situation, and an enhanced involvement in their treatment. Several studies have specifically examined coping strategies of HIV-positive gay men. With a sample of twenty-nine men Wolf and colleagues (1991) found that active coping was associated with enhanced mood and negatively related to a global measure of psychological distress. Avoidance was significantly related to depression. Nicholson and Long (1990) also noted negative effects of avoidant coping. In their sample of eighty-nine HIV-positive gay men, an avoidant style was associated with a diminished self-view. These results all point to the same conclusion: active, problem-focused coping is an effective mechanism for enhancing mood in terminally ill patients. In addition, these strategies may lead to problem resolution and an enhanced sense of mastery and control. Thus they should be a significant focus of treatment with this population.

In addition to teaching problem-solving and cognitive restructuring skills, treatment must address meaning and spirituality. A thorough case conceptualization is necessary so that the meaning of the dying can be understood within the framework of the person's entire life experiences. The patient may want to review prior experiences, both positive and negative, to determine significant personal themes or gain a new understanding of his or her identity. This review may lead the patient to define certain accomplishments he or she would still like to achieve (Feigenberg 1975). Certain unfulfilled goals may have to be acknowledged and reconciled. For example, a patient who has a distant relationship with a parent may choose to try and resolve past disputes or accept that this cannot be changed and thus direct attention to other significant relationships. The therapist can help the patient prioritize his or her goals and realistically assess what can be accomplished in the remaining time. Reframing lost opportunities is also possible. Focusing on what the person has achieved and modifying the significance of the unaccomplished may make the resolution easier.

In addition to finding meaning in the life that was lived, the patient may try to find meaning in death. Answering "Why me?" may become an important goal for the patient. The therapist should not impose a meaning for the patient but can facilitate an answer by having the patient discuss his or her interpretation of why this occurred. The therapist should intervene, however, if the rationale is self- or other-deprecating or results in despair. If the patient's explanation leads to distress, the therapist can help him or her develop an alternative by asking such questions as "What's another way of looking at it?" "How would (a significant other) explain this?" "What is the evidence for this (negative) explanation?" Reframing the meaning so that the patient finds an acceptable and calming interpretation may thus become a focus of treatment.

Patients may turn to a personal philosophy or religious system to construe meaning (Gibbs and Achterberg-Lawlis 1978). The therapist must accept this interpretation without adding his or her own beliefs (Smith et al. 1983). The goal is to help the patient clarify and perhaps redefine his or her belief system so that it is a source of comfort. The content that the patient develops is less significant than the actual process of defining these views.

Enhancing control and a sense of meaning are prominent therapy goals with patients dying of AIDS. It is clear that addressing these concerns can diminish distress. An added benefit is that the techniques outlined here can help with other problematic situations and serve as general adaptive strategies.

Alleviating Fears of Pain

Fear of the dying process, as well as the fear of death, may be a significant concern. Two categories of concern are particularly salient: fear of the unknown and fear of pain. Uncertainty about disease progression, future treatment, and available care may lead to overwhelming anxiety (Sherr 1989a). To address these issues, patients must be taught to specifically identify their concerns, develop questions to elicit information, and direct the questions to the appropriate sources. This communication may clarify ambiguous aspects and enhance understanding. Discussing viable options may produce a sense of certainty and relief.

Pain management is another prominent concern of dying AIDS patients. Fishman (1992) argues that it is essential that patients be taught the distinction between pain, a sensory stimulus, and suffering, an experience that reflects threatening beliefs. Patients must learn that their beliefs affect their emotions and subsequent physical sensations. The assumption that they will not be able to control their pain heightens arousal and thus increases the unpleasant sensation. Teaching patients specific strategies to enhance their pain control and modify their thoughts will produce a sense of mastery as well as diminish pain sensations.

AIDS patients have specific constellations of noteworthy symptoms. AIDS dementia represents the most frequent neurological diagnosis in this population (Tross and Hirsch 1988); two-thirds of patients develop this complex. It is caused by an infection to the brain and is marked by widespread and complete cognitive deterioration. Patients often fear developing dementia and may react with great anxiety or depression as they begin to notice cognitive impairment. Moynihan and colleagues (1988) recommend that these possibilities and concerns be addressed directly with the patient. It is important to emphasize which of the symptoms can be modified by treatment. Planning ahead and deciding who will assume control if the patient becomes cognitively impaired might allay some concerns about responsibility and safety.

The therapist must be alert to symptoms that might suggest dementia is developing. Changes in mood, speech, or motor functioning may indicate neurological damage. Affective changes may reflect organic causes; clinicians must not assume that all mood symptoms are due to psychological distress (Tross and Hirsch 1988). The therapist may need to become involved with making referrals to appropriate medical specialists and should be aware of the resources available in the community.

The Final Phase of Therapy

The most challenging aspect of psychotherapy with patients dying of AIDS may be when they are closest to death. The patient may realize that he or she will soon die. Hope and denial may cease and resignation predominate (Lomax and Sandler 1988). The patient should be reminded that his or her previous decisions about treatment will be respected. Ensuring that pain management and daily care needs are met are also priorities (Markowitz et al. 1994). Changes in mental status must be monitored to assess both mood and cognitive deterioration. Patients may be at increased risk for suicide. Legally, the therapist cannot support this option. Patients may view suicide as a method to control their pain and deterioration. The therapist can discuss these issues, but is prevented by the law from aiding the patient in taking his/her life (Lomax and Sandler 1988).

As cognitive abilities decline, standard therapy may be difficult or impossible to continue. However, the therapist should continue to be available through phone calls or brief visits

(Feigenberg 1975, Lomax and Sandler 1988). This contact may continue to be a valuable resource to the patient. The therapist should also maintain contact with the medical staff and family to see that the patient's wishes are honored and to provide support to the loved ones.

This section has examined treatment with patients dying of AIDS. Certain themes and diverse techniques may be shared across patients. However, the most important caveat is individual case conceptualization. The therapist must not assume that particular issues and interventions are relevant for all patients. A flexible view must guide treatment so that the needs of the individual are best served.

Family Issues and Treatment

Most people do not die of AIDS in isolation. Loved ones are a significant aspect of the process and their needs and concerns must be addressed. Watching a loved one die of AIDS is associated with several unique factors (Stulberg and Buckingham 1988). Families may have just recently learned of the patient's lifestyle and may have difficulty accepting it. It may be awkward or uncomfortable for them to see the patient with his lover, particularly as they come together to visit the patient or make treatment decisions. Families may keep the patient's diagnosis private because of shame or fear of rejection and thus deprive themselves of sources of support. In addition, lying or not disclosing the diagnosis may lead to a fear of being uncovered or anger that disclosure would not be accepted. They may feel guilty if they assume they are responsible for the patient's homosexuality or drug use. Finally, the loss of a child counters parents' expectations and hopes for the future. Parents expect that their offspring will outlive them; this assumption is shattered as the patient deteriorates (Worden 1991).

Power struggles may develop as the person weakens. The

loved ones may want to protect the patient but inadvertently take away tasks he or she is still capable of performing (Frierson et al. 1987). Others may not recognize the severity of the patient's health and make impossible demands, while not offering support (Moynihan et al. 1988). Maintaining a balance between fostering the patient's autonomy and guaranteeing that needs are met is a goal that should guide the family's actions.

Observing the physical deterioration may be tremendously distressing (Worden 1991). The unpredictable course of the illness may lead to a sense of helplessness and uncontrollability in loved ones (Frierson et al. 1987). Gradually, the inevitability of death can no longer be denied or avoided. It may become increasingly painful to be near the patient. Furthermore, as the patient changes so drastically, it may be difficult to retain positive images of how he or she was prior to the illness.

A variety of specific stressors are associated with being a gay male whose partner is dying of AIDS. The relationship may be viewed as a marriage by the couple, but not by social and legal structures (Murphy and Perry 1988). Thus the lover does not have the rights of a heterosexual spouse. The partner may be barred from hospital visits, be permitted only limited time away from work, not be involved with treatment or funeral decisions, and have no inheritance rights (Barrows and Halgin 1988). If the partner is not open about his sexuality, he may have limited opportunities for support and feel isolated (Biller and Rice 1990, Pheifer and Houseman 1988, Siegal and Hoefer 1981). The partner may have his own health concerns and vulnerabilities. He may be HIV-positive or fear contracting the virus. Guilt may be prevalent if the partner gave the virus to the patient (Worden 1991). He may also be concerned about who will care for him if he becomes sick in the future (Sherr et al. 1992). The age of the lover may mean that he has limited experience coping with death. However, it is also possible that the partner is experiencing bereavement overload if he knows many others in the community who are also sick or deceased (Dean et al. 1988). Even if the partner has many support resources, these friends may be mourning other losses and thus be unable to be of much assistance (Barrows and Halgin 1988).

Loved ones who serve as caretakers face additional challenges. Pearlin and colleagues (1988) suggest that caretakers have three stressors: the actual caregiving role, personal health concerns, and additional life strains. Meeting the needs of a person dying of AIDS can be extraordinarily draining. Demands heighten as the patient declines and the caregiver may become increasingly overwhelmed. Duties are all-encompassing and time consuming. Multiple and diverse roles must be assumed, including friend, nurse, therapist, and liaison. The second stressor may be the caregiver's own uncertain health. If the provider is HIV-positive, he or she may fear dying in a similar painful manner. The caregiver may also be concerned that no one will be able to give care to him or her when it becomes necessary. Finally, the caregiving role invades all areas of one's life and may create additional difficulties. For example, job performance or security might suffer, other relationships are disregarded, and financial resources depleted. If the provider does try to attend to other life areas, the quality of the caregiving might be compromised. The caregiver faces a tremendous dilemma in trying to prioritize his or her responsibilities.

One study (Trice 1988) has examined the toll of caregiving to dying AIDS patients. Forty-three mothers were interviewed two to three years after their sons died from AIDS. Eighty-four percent of the women who had served as full-time caregivers showed symptoms of post-traumatic stress disorder. In addition, they reported elevated rates of marital separation or divorce, job changes, night terrors, aggression, panic attacks, migraine headaches, and hypertension. This research demonstrates the extent to which caregiving can have negative sequelae.

Other work has examined the impact of having a close loved one die from AIDS, independent of caretaking responsibilities. Martin and Dean (1993; see also Martin 1988) utilized a sample of 746 gay men, followed for up to seven years. The bereaved reported greater rates of psychological distress than the non-bereaved, particularly traumatic stress response symptoms. The highest levels of distress were found in subjects who were HIV-positive or had AIDS as well as being bereaved. Within one to two years of the loss, psychological symptoms diminished. This suggests that although loss may be initially distressing, the bereaved may experience fewer symptoms over time. Neugebauer and colleagues (1992) reported on a sample of 207 gay men. They did not find a relationship between number of losses and depression. However, bereavement distress, or a preoccupation with and yearning for the loved one, was correlated with number of losses. Thus, while loss did not cause depression in this sample, it was associated with other symptoms of distress. Lennon and colleagues (1990) summarize their work by concluding that grief reactions among gay men are similar to those reported by heterosexual spouses. However, the symptoms were associated with caretaking responsibilities and perceived inadequacy of social support. This suggests that clinicians should not examine bereavement responses in isolation but must also attend to precipitating or additional stressors.

The previous section discussed the negative impact of experiencing a loved one's dying of AIDS. Intervention may be necessary for coping with the patient's dying, after the death occurs, or at both points. Individuals within a family may respond very differently. The therapist must be aware of two systems: the overall family dynamics and each member's coping style (Rainey 1988). The clinician might first have contact with the family as the patient's individual therapist. Sherr (1989b) recommends that the therapist should also attend to the family's role and involve them in the treatment, when appropriate.

Frierson and colleagues (1987) have outlined several themes that should be incorporated when working with families. Of primary importance is assessing whether the family has accurate information about AIDS. Answering questions, correcting misinformation, and providing appropriate resources will enhance understanding, clarify ambiguities, and diminish uncertainty. These researchers argue that some individuals may be denying certain aspects of the illness and recommend that protective denial not be questioned if it is not creating additional stressors. They also emphasize the utilization of support groups so that family members can use others as a source of support as well as coping models in a nonjudgmental environment. Murphy and Perry (1988) outline a short-term support group intervention. They believe the leader should primarily have a supportive and educative role: teaching about grief, normalizing the response, and emphasizing individual variation.

Others (Pearlin et al. 1988) have addressed more general therapeutic strategies for loved ones. Cognitive and behavioral techniques may be useful for controlling mood and keeping stressors from becoming too overwhelming. For example, a parent who believes that he or she must keep the child's illness a secret can be taught to rationally examine this belief and its associated behaviors. The parent can be taught how to pick appropriate people to confide in as well as ways to discuss the issues more comfortably. If a family member feels overwhelmed by caretaking duties, he or she can learn how to schedule time differently or assertively ask others to help.

Different therapeutic interventions for the family may become necessary after the patient dies. Pheifer and Houseman (1988) outline factors that should be incorporated when working with the bereaved. The mourner may be encouraged to identify and express the varied emotions he or she is experiencing. These reactions should be normalized so that the individual does not feel different or inadequate. A new life without the loved one will have to be developed. The mourner will have to begin to turn to others for needs the deceased previously fulfilled. A didactic component of treatment may be necessary if the bereaved has certain faulty beliefs about the time-course or emotions of bereavement. Evaluating coping styles and teaching alternatives may be recommended if the mourner is in great distress or if his or her style is ineffective.

Schwartzberg (1992) argues that models of grief are particularly inadequate for gay men and new theories must be developed that can incorporate the impact of ongoing multiple deaths, features of gay male culture, and finding meaning in loss. Existing models are inappropriate because gay men have experienced numerous losses, encompassing their support network and extended community. In addition, the illness is stigmatized and these men might be facing their own impending death. Schwartzberg stresses that finding meaning is paramount for the bereaved. Mourners might try to achieve this through political, community, or spiritual involvement. Issues of living in a world without meaning might also develop in therapy. Subsequently, an enhanced sense of vulnerability or despair may occur. Developing alternative views of the world or ways to find meaning and satisfaction may become a therapeutic issue.

This final section has delineated the concerns of family members of dying AIDS patients. While the general bereavement literature is a useful guide, special considerations for AIDS must be noted. The youth of the patient, the stigmatization of the illness, and personal health concerns of loved ones are factors that have generally not been considered in other illnesses. Despite these additional features, previously developed therapeutic interventions can be applied successfully. Normalizing the grief reaction, helping to find meaning, and teaching cognitive and behavioral coping strategies all contribute to diminishing the distress of the bereaved.

REFERENCES

Barrows, P. A., and Halgin, R. P. (1988). Current issues in psychotherapy with gay men: impact of the AIDS phenomenon. *Professional Psychology: Research and Practice* 19:395–402.

Biller, R., and Rice, S. (1990). Experiencing multiple loss of persons with AIDS: grief and bereavement issues. *Health and Social Work* 15:283–290.

Carey, R. G. (1974). Emotional adjustment in terminal patients: a quantitative approach. *Journal of Counseling Psychology* 21:433–439.

Corr, C. A. (1991). A task-based approach to coping with dying. *Omega* 24:81–94.

——— (1993). Coping with dying: lessons that we should and should not learn from the work of Elizabeth Kubler-Ross. *Death Studies* 17:69–83.

Dean, L., Hall, W. E., and Martin, J. L. (1988). Chronic and intermittent AIDS related bereavement in a panel of homosexual men in New York City. *Journal of Palliative Care* 4:54–57.

Feifel, H., and Branscomb, A. B. (1981). Who's afraid of death? *Journal of Abnormal Psychology* 81:282–288.

Fiefel, H., Strack, S., and Nagy, V. T. (1987). Degree of life-threat and differential use of coping modes. *Journal of Psychosomatic Research* 31:91–99.

Feigenberg, L. (1975). Care and understanding of the dying: a patient-centered approach. *Omega* 6:81–94.

Fishman, B. (1992). The cognitive-behavioral perspective on pain management in terminal illness. *The Hospice Journal* 8:73–88.

Frierson, R. L., Lippmann, S. B., and Johnson, J. (1987). AIDS: psychological stresses on the family. *Psychosomatics* 28:65–68.

Gibbs, H. W., and Achterberg-Lawlis, J. (1978). Spiritual values and death anxiety: implications for counseling with terminal patients. *Journal of Counseling Psychology* 25:563–569.

Hintze, J., Templer, D. I., Cappelletty, G. G., and Frederick, W. (1994). Death depression and death anxiety in HIV-infected males. In *Death Anxiety Handbook*, ed. R. Neimeyer, pp. 193–200. Washington, DC: Taylor and Francis.

Kelly, J. A., and Murphy, D. A. (1992). Psychological interventions with AIDS and HIV: prevention and treatment. *Journal of Consulting and Clinical Psychology* 60:576–585.

Kelly, J. A., and St. Lawrence, J. S. (1988). AIDS prevention and treatment: psychology's role in the health crisis. *Clinical Psychology Review* 8:255–284.

Lennon, M. C., Martin, J. L., and Dean, L. (1990). The influence of social support on AIDS-related grief reactions among gay men. *Social Science Medicine* 31:477–484.

Lomax, G. L., and Sandler, J. (1988). Psychotherapy and consultation with persons with AIDS. *Psychiatric Annals* 18:253–259.

Markowitz, J. C., Rabkin, J. G., and Perry, S. W. (1994). Treating depression in HIV-positive patients. *AIDS* 8:403–412.

Martin, J. L. (1988). Psychological consequences of AIDS-related bereavement among gay men. *Journal of Consulting and Clinical Psychology* 56:856–862.

Martin, J. L., and Dean, L. (1993). Effects of AIDS-related bereavement and HIV-related illness on psychological distress among gay men: a seven-year longitudinal study, 1985–1991. *Journal of Consulting and Clinical Psychology* 61:94–103.

McKusick, L. (1988). The impact of AIDS on practitioner and client: notes for the therapeutic relationship. *American Psychologist* 43:935–940.

Morgan, J. D. (1988). Living our dying: social and cultural considerations. In *Dying: Facing the Facts*, ed. H. Wass, F. M. Burardo, and R. A. Neimeyer, pp. 13–27. Washington, DC: Hemisphere.

Moynihan, R., Christ, G., and Silver, L. G. (1988). AIDS and terminal illness. *Social Casework* 69:380–387.

Murphy, P., and Perry, K. (1988). Hidden grievers. *Death Studies* 12:451–462.

Naysmith, A., and O'Neill, W. (1989). Hospice. In *Death, Dying, and Bereavement*, ed. L. Sherr, pp. 1–16. Oxford: Blackwell.

Neugebauer, R., Rabkin, J. G., Williams, J. B. W., et al. (1992).

Bereavement reactions among homosexual men experiencing multiple losses in the AIDS epidemic. *American Journal of Psychiatry* 149:1374–1379.

Nicholson, W. D., and Long, B. C. (1990). Self-esteem, social support, internalized homophobia, and coping strategies of HIV-positive gay men. *Journal of Consulting and Clinical Psychology* 58:873–876.

Pearlin, L. I., Semple, S., and Turner, H. (1988). Stress of AIDS caregiving: a preliminary overview of the issues. *Death Studies* 12:501–517.

Pheifer, W. G., and Houseman, C. (1988). Bereavement and AIDS: a framework for intervention. *Journal of Psychosocial Nursing* 26:21–26.

Rainey, R. C. (1988). The Experience of Dying. In *Dying: Facing the Facts*, ed. H. Wass, F. M. Berardo, and R. A. Neimeyer, pp. 137–157. Washington, DC: Hemisphere.

Schulz, R., and Aderman, D. (1974). Clinical research and the stages of dying. *Omega* 5:137–143.

Schwartzberg, S. S. (1992). AIDS-related bereavement among gay men: the inadequacy of current theories of grief. *Psychotherapy* 29:422–429.

Sherr, L. (1989a). AIDS. In *Death, Dying, and Bereavement*, ed. L. Sherr, pp. 179–196. Oxford: Blackwell.

——— (1989b). Staff training - a necessity, not a luxury. In *Death, Dying, and Bereavement*, ed. L. Sherr, pp. 48–67. Oxford: Blackwell.

Sherr, L., Hedge, B., Steinhart, K., et al. (1992). Unique patterns of bereavement in HIV: implications for counselling. *Genitourinary Medicine* 68:378–381.

Siegal, R. L., and Hoefer, D. D. (1981). Bereavement counseling for gay individuals. *American Journal of Psychotherapy* 35:517–525.

Smith, D. K., Nehemkis, A. M., and Charter, R. A. (1983). Fear of death, death attitudes, and religious conviction in the terminally ill. *International Journal of Psychiatry* 13:221–232.

Speck, P. (1989). Cultural and religious aspects of dying. In *Death, Dying, and Bereavement*, ed. L. Sherr, pp. 36–47. Oxford: Blackwell.

Stulberg, I., and Buckingham, S. L. (1988). Parallel issues for AIDS patients, families, and others. *Social Casework* 69:355–359.

Taylor, S. E. (1983). Adjustment to threatening events: a theory of cognitive adaptation. *American Psychologist* 38:1161–1173.

Tomer, A. (1994). Death anxiety in adult life - theoretical perspectives. In *Death Anxiety Handbook: Research, Instrumentation, and Application*, ed. R. A. Neimeyer, pp. 3–28. Washington, DC: Taylor and Francis.

Trice, A. D. (1988). Post-traumatic stress syndrome-like symptoms among AIDS caregivers. *Psychological Reports* 63:656–658.

Tross, S., and Hirsch, D. A. (1988). Psychological distress and neuropsychological complications of HIV infection and AIDS. *American Psychologist* 43:929–934.

Weisman, A. D., and Worden, J. W. (1976). The existential plight in cancer: significance of the first 100 days. *International Journal of Psychiatry in Medicine* 7:1–15.

Wolf, T. M., Balson, P. M., Morse, E. V., et al. (1991). Relationship of coping style to affective state and perceived social support in asymptomatic and symptomatic HIV-infected persons: implications for clinical management. *Journal of Clinical Psychiatry* 52:171–173.

Wong, P. T. P., Reker, G. T., and Gesser, G. (1994). Death Attitude Profile-Revised: A Multidimensional Measure of Attitudes Toward Death. In *Death Anxiety Handbook: Research, Instrumentation, and Application*, ed. R. Neimeyer, pp. 121–148. Washington, DC: Taylor and Francis.

Worden, J. W. (1991). Grieving a loss from AIDS. *Hospice Journal* 7:143–150.

5

HIV Disease and African-American Gay and Bisexual Men

ISIAAH CRAWFORD

We are now well into our second decade of contending with the medical and psychosocial ramifications of HIV. The impact that it has had upon the African-American community has been severe and unrelenting. Although African-Americans constitute only 12 percent of the United States population, they represent over 30 percent of all individuals diagnosed with HIV disease. In 1994, African-American men who identified themselves as "men who have sex with men" accounted for 23 percent of the newly diagnosed cases of AIDS (Centers for Disease Control and Prevention [CDC] 1995). Women with AIDS are overwhelmingly African-American (53 percent), and over 60 percent of pediatric AIDS cases are also found within this community (CDC 1995). These figures are a sobering demonstration of the pervasive impact HIV is currently having upon the African-American community and is poised to have for many years to come.

Faced with the historical, social, and economic hurdles that accompany ethnic minority status in the United States, many urban African-Americans now find themselves having to combat the physical and emotional devastation caused by a life-threatening illness. The stress this imposes upon an individual's internal and external support systems is often overwhelming. As discussed in Chapter 1, the medical stages of HIV infection carry concurrent psychological reactions and sequelae. Although each stage or medical event of the illness is accompanied by emotional challenges and stressors that are universal, the manner in which they manifest themselves often varies across specific individuals and ethnic racial groups. Understanding the social and cultural context of HIV, sexuality, and identity development within the African-American community is essential before one can lend psychotherapeutic support to an HIV-impacted gay or bisexual African-American male. The intent of this chapter is to present a conceptual model that details not only the common emotional experiences of individuals as they progress through the medical course of HIV disease, but also to reveal how these experiences may differ for African-American gay and bisexual men. In addition, the narrative outlines psychotherapeutic strategies that mental health providers can consider using in their work with these HIV-infected African-Americans.

THE CULTURAL CONTEXT OF HIV

Before we progress in our discussion of the emotional ramifications of HIV infection and suggested treatment strategies, it seems prudent to address several cultural issues that should be considered in providing care to African-American gay and bisexual men. The issues that demand the sensitive understanding and appreciation of mental health professionals include (1) the sexual attitudes of the African-American community, (2) cultural mistrust, and (3) racial and sexual identity development. These factors are interwoven in how African-American gay and bisexual men conceptualize HIV, respond to its threat, and cope with its infection.

Sexual Attitudes of the African-American Community

The scant amount of psychological research on the attitudes of African-Americans toward homosexuality suggests that, as a group, most possess traditional religious views and consequently have a very negative outlook upon same-gender sexual activity (Greene 1994, Herek and Capitanio 1995, Michael et al. 1994). Sexual behavior of this nature is perceived as sinful and unnatural, and individuals known to engage in this activity should be counseled and urged to stop. Otherwise, they face a terrible consequence: eternal damnation.

Herek and Capitanio (1995) report from their national telephone survey of African-Americans that African-American heterosexual men hold a somewhat more negative attitude toward gay men than do African-American women, primarily because of the greater likelihood for men to regard homosexuality as unnatural. Their findings also indicate that African-Americans who believe homosexuality is something within the control of an individual are more likely to hold negative and uncompromising attitudes toward homosexuality (Herek and Capitanio 1995).

It has been noted that at some level there is an acceptance of homosexuality in African-American communities; however, this tolerance comes with the undocumented agreement that gay and bisexual African-Americans must not disclose their sexual orientations or display "obvious" signs of their sexual identities (Dalton 1989, Mays 1989, Peterson 1992). As long as they do not confront the community with their lifestyles, gay and bisexual African-Americans will be accepted. Leonard Paterson (1983) writes that this dynamic is often seen in the African-American church, where many gay and bisexual men are often positioned prominently; however, significant aspects of their lives are maintained in secrecy to protect their status within the community. For others within the community, homosexuality is viewed as a threat to the survival of African-Americans within the United States. Gay and lesbian African-Americans are seen as unwittingly contributing to the demise of the

African-American family structure. Gay African-American males are perceived to be rejecting African-American women; consequently, a pool of promising young African-Americans are not marrying and producing offspring who can contribute to the mission of the community.

Although this discussion of the underpinnings of homophobia within the African-American community is largely theoretical in nature, it warrants consideration for it demonstrates the complexity of the issue. Moreover, it displays what the African-American gay and bisexual male is challenged by within the African-American community. What we discern is that gay and bisexual African-American men are confronted with the fear of being rejected, demeaned, and ostracized by their community if their sexual orientation is discovered. What has allowed African-Americans to survive years of discrimination and bigotry within this country has been the strength of the African-American church and its clergy, and the willingness of the members of the African-American community to support one another. Maintaining a sense of cohesion and connectedness with the community is an essential emotional requirement for many African-Americans (Akbar 1984, Jones and Block 1984). Experiencing feelings of communal detachment and isolation are often associated with increased levels of physical and emotional dysfunction among African-Americans (Chimezie 1985). Facing the threat of social and emotional abandonment, many gay and bisexual black men are challenged to maintain a dual existence that often has significant psychological consequences (Greene 1994).

For some, this means leading a compartmentalized existence. Recognizing that only a part of oneself is valued within the African-American community, the gay and bisexual African-American male must monitor and measure what he reveals, while simultaneously seeking out the white gay community for the expression of the other aspects of his identity. Others may choose to leave the community completely and seek refuge in the gay community; however, this coping strategy is also fraught with emotional hazards. The white gay community possesses the same bigotry and biases of the general white community. Even within this community, the African-American gay and bisexual male is not likely to experience complete acceptance and understanding.

Existence as a gay or bisexual African-American male in American society is extremely challenging. It is crucial for the mental health provider to be sensitive to the factors that contribute to this struggle. How the gay or bisexual African-American male living with AIDS navigates these issues is of profound importance to his ability to cope with the medical and psychological effects of the disease syndrome.

Cultural Mistrust of Public Health Information and Interventions

The history of slavery and racism in this country has played a significant role in developing the current social environment many African-Americans encounter. The aspirations engendered by the civil rights movement of the 1960s have not been realized for the vast majority. African-Americans' consequent anger and despair in the face of persistent inequality have contributed to the development of conspiracy theories about Caucasians (i.e., the government) against African-Americans (Thomas and Quinn 1991). These theories range from the belief that the government promotes drug abuse in the African-American community to the belief that HIV is a man-made weapon of racial warfare (Thomas and Quinn 1991).

As cited by Thomas and Quinn (1991), the Nation of Islam and mainstream African-American media (e.g., *Essence Magazine, The Los Angeles Sentinel,* and *Tony Brown's Journal*) have broadcast and written material suggesting that AIDS is a form of genocide to destroy the Negro race. This, coupled with the saga of the Tuskegee Syphilis Study that involved the failure to inform and adequately treat African-American participants, has helped to breed the current pervasive sense of distrust toward public health officials and institutionalized medicine and science.

In 1990, the Southern Christian Leadership Conference (SCLC), a leading civil rights organization, received funding from the CDC to provide HIV education through a national program entitled Reducing AIDS through Community Education. To determine the HIV education needs in the African-American community, the SCLC surveyed 1,056 African-American church members in five cities. The results of their needs assessment revealed that 35 percent of the respondents believed that AIDS is a form of genocide; another 30 percent were unsure. Moreover, 44 percent believed the government is withholding information (i.e., the "truth") about AIDS, and 34 percent believed that AIDS is man-made (as cited in Thomas and Quinn 1991).

Mistrust of this nature creates an additional barrier in the prevention and treatment of HIV disease. Suspiciousness and apprehension toward the medical and scientific communities lead many African-Americans to be reluctant to receive prophylactic care, follow treatment protocols, or participate in clinical research trials for fear of being victimized further by a malevolent system. Many AIDS service organizations are located outside the African-American community, and lack a multicultural focus in their staffing, physical plant, or educational materials. All these factors have contributed to the resistance of African-Americans to pay attention to health promotion information or to seek out available services.

Mental health professionals working with African-American gay and bisexual males must keep the aforementioned concerns in mind as they attempt to develop a working alliance with their patients. Establishing rapport and developing trust within these relationships must be done with a great deal of fidelity. It is important for the service provider to remember that he/she represents a medical and scientific community that has a scandalous reputation to overcome among many African-Americans.

Racial and Sexual Identity Development

The most basic aspect of human awareness centers on the question "Who am I?" Seeking self-understanding, a clarity of personhood, is one of our most primary instincts. Arriving at an answer to this universal question that allows one to feel a sense of personal value and esteem is often viewed as an essential element for good mental health. For the African-American gay or bisexual male, this process can be a very complex and treacherous undertaking. In Western society, what is not Caucasian and not heterosexual has historically not been valued or celebrated. In fact, it has often been denigrated and demeaned. The impact of this devaluation upon the identity development of gay or bisexual African-Americans is often substantial. To work effectively with this population, mental health professionals must become cognizant of the unique identity development process that racial-ethnic and sexual minorities undergo within this culture. To assist the reader, a conceptual model of minority identity development is presented in this chapter, followed by a more specific formulation related to gay identity development.

Several theorists have discussed how the process of identity development for individuals of minority status differs from that of their majority counterparts (Carney and Kahn 1984, Cross 1971, Helms 1993, Parham 1981, Ponterotto 1988, Ruiz and Padilla 1977). Atkinson and colleagues (1989) have drawn parallels across racial-ethnic groups, gays and lesbians, women, and disabled persons and have noted that the common experience of oppression serves as a unifying factor in the identity development of individuals belonging to these diverse minority groups. It is their belief that as minority individuals become increasingly aware of themselves as objects of oppression, their attitudes toward themselves, their own minority groups, other minority groups, and members of the dominant culture evolve in a systematic manner that leads to a core sense of identity. This premise is supported by the pervasive number of existing societal "isms" (racism, sexism, and ageism) and their impact on those whom society at large (i.e., majority culture) would define as inferior (Myers et al. 1991). Atkinson and colleagues (1989) constructed a paradigm, the Minority Identity Development model (MID), that outlines the attitudinal processes and shifts, and corresponding behaviors, that follow a five-stage sequence. Atkinson and his colleagues do not perceive the MID as a comprehensive theory of personality development, but rather as a schema to assist mental health professionals in understanding minority clients within existing personality frameworks. The authors are clear in their discussion that although the MID consists of five distinct stages, it is more accurately conceptualized as a continuous process in which one stage blends with another and boundaries between stages are fluid. Table 5–1 is a description of the MID.

Table 5–1. Summary Minority Identity Development Model

Stages of Minority Development Model	Attitude toward Self	Attitude toward others of the same minority	Attitude toward others of different minority	Attitude toward dominant group
Stage 1 — Conformity	self-deprecating	group-deprecating	discriminatory	group-appreciation
Stage 2 — Dissonance	conflict between self-deprecating and appreciating	conflict between group-deprecating and group-appreciating	conflict between dominant-held views of minority hierarchy and feelings of shared experience	conflict between group-appreciating and group-deprecating
Stage 3 — Resistance and immersion	self-appreciation	group-appreciation	conflict between feelings of empathy for other minority experiences and feelings of cultural-centrism	group-deprecating
Stage 4 — Introspection	concern with basis of self-appreciation	concern with nature of unequivocal appreciation	concern with ethnocentric basis for judging others	concern with the basis of group deprecation
Stage 5 — Synergetic Articulation and Awareness	self-appreciating	group-appreciating	group-appreciating	selective-appreciation

Stage 1: Conformity

Minority individuals in this stage of development hold an unequivocal preference and idealization toward the dominant culture and its values over those of their own culture. Their choices of role models, lifestyles, and value systems are all in accord with the dominant group. Physical or cultural traits that identify them as minority persons are abhorred, held in contempt, and often repressed (Atkinson et al. 1989). Consequently, minority individuals in this stage view themselves, fellow group members, and other minorities with disdain, devaluation, and often intense negativity. These individuals are strongly driven to assimilate and acculturate into the dominant culture and to distance themselves from their minority culture and heritage as much as possible. Negative stereotypes of their minority group are believed, other minority groups are viewed from the dominant group's perspective, and minority groups that resemble the majority culture are viewed more favorably.

In this Conformity Stage, minorities view themselves as deficient in "desirable" attributes held up by the dominant society. Feelings of racial self-hatred characterize this individual's self-identity.

Stage 2: Dissonance

The second stage is marked by gradual awareness of minority cultural strengths. This awareness is stimulated primarily when the individual is confronted by situations or events that conflict with the negative beliefs that the individual holds toward his own minority group. To elucidate this phenomenon, Atkinson and colleagues (1989) provide an example of an encounter between an African-American male who feels ashamed of his cultural history and upbringing and an African-American who seems proud of his cultural heritage. The former is now in a position of having to rethink his beliefs. The type of feelings that correspond with this state are alternating emotions of shame and pride in the self. Values and attitudes of the dominant culture are now called into question as new, inconsistent information is received indicating that not all majority culture values are beneficial for individuals of minority status. Cultural values of the minority group begin to have appeal and feelings of alliance with oppressed people develop (Atkinson et al. 1989).

Stage 3: Resistance and Immersion

The third stage, Resistance and Immersion, represents an almost complete reformulation on the part of the minority individual. The individual now completely endorses minority-held views and rejects the dominant society and culture. A desire to eliminate oppression of the individual's minority group becomes an important motivation of the individual's behavior (Atkinson et al. 1989). This transformation seems to be motivated by two primary factors. First, the individual has been able to resolve many of the conflicts that were present during the Dissonance Stage; consequently, a greater appreciation for the societal forces of racism, oppression, and discrimination emerges, along with the realization that he/she has been victimized by it (Sue and Sue 1990). Concomitantly, intense feelings of guilt, shame, and anger have been stimulated. The feelings of guilt and shame arise from the sense that the individual had "sold out" in the past and contributed to his or her own group's oppression; the feelings of anger arise from the individual's having been victimized and "converted" by the forces of the dominant group.

African-American males in this stage of development are exploring their history and culture, seeking out information that will enhance their sense of identity. Cultural and physical attributes that once incited feelings of self-loathing and recrimination are now perceived as symbols of pride and honor (Atkinson et al. 1989). Attitudes toward members of the same minority group are idealized and cultural values of this group are accepted without question.

Stage 4: Introspection

The African-American male in the Introspection Stage is confronting feelings of discontent and discomfort with group views rigidly held in the Resistance and Immersion Stage, and diverts attention to notions of greater individual autonomy (Atkinson et al. 1989). The authors contend that the minority individual has begun to feel more comfortable with his own sense of identity; consequently, he is able to question the beliefs of the Resistance Stage that all Caucasians and their values are without merit. What seems to characterize this stage is that greater individual autonomy is present, yet uneasiness exists with regard to how that may conflict with minority group allegiance (Atkinson et al. 1989).

Stage 5: Synergetic Articulation and Awareness

The African-American male in this stage possesses an integrated sense of self-identity. He is characterized by a strong sense of self-worth, confidence, and autonomy, the result of his establishing an identity as an individual, a member of a minority group, and a member of the larger society. He possesses a sense of pride in his minority group without having to accept group values without question. Concurrently, he has respect for and supports members of other minority groups and he selectively trusts and likes members of the dominant group (Atkinson et al. 1989). Conflicts and discomforts of the previous stage have been resolved, allowing greater individual control and autonomy. Cultural values of other minorities as well as those of the dominant group are objectively examined and accepted or rejected on the basis of experience gained in earlier stages of identity development (Atkinson et al. 1989). For many, the desire to eliminate all forms of oppression becomes a salient component in their outlook on life.

This model is presented as a framework to assist the mental

health professional in conceptualizing the issues surrounding minority identity development. It should be noted that all minority individuals do not progress through all of the aforementioned stages, and they may vacillate between stages at different points in their lives. Although the model is not absolute, it does provide a way for mental health professionals to begin to better understand the role of oppression and racism and to appreciate the within-group variation that exists among members of the same racial-ethnic minority group (i.e., African-American).

Not only does the African-American gay or bisexual male have to contend with the developmental process of his racial-ethnic identity, he is also confronted with an additional developmental challenge—sexual identity, as elaborated in the following discussion of the most contemporary formulation of this process.

The Process of Sexual Identity Formation

One of the most well-received and accepted models of sexual identity formulation has been conceptualized by Richard Troiden (1993). He has synthesized the work of many individuals over the last 25 years (Cass 1979, 1984, Coleman 1982, Lee 1977, Ponse 1978, Schäfer 1976, Weinberg 1978) with his own (Troiden 1979), which incorporates the results of research investigating the coming-out process of gay men and lesbians. Troiden views sexual identity as something that is internalized into one's self-concept (i.e., mental image) similarly to other aspects of one's identity, such as gender or racial-ethnic heritage. It is Troiden's belief that a perception of the self as homosexual is an attitude, a potential line of action toward the self and others that is mobilized in settings—imagined or real—defined as sexual, romantic, or social in nature (Troiden 1993). Vivienne Cass (1979, 1984) believes that the homosexual identity may function as a self-identity, a perceived identity, a presented identity, or a combination of all three, depending on contextual factors. From this perspective the homosexual identity can be conceptualized as a self-identity when people view themselves as homosexual in relation to romantic and sexual situations. It can be construed as a perceived identity in situations in which people think or know that others view them as homosexual. It is a presented identity when people present or announce themselves as homosexual in general social settings.

The contemporary line of reasoning holds that when the self-identity, perceived identity, and presented identities exist concurrently, the homosexual individual is most integrated because an agreement exists between who people think they are, who they claim they are, and how others view them. How one manages to synthesize these aspects of his/her sexual identity is conceptualized as a series of stages that one moves through in gay or bisexual identity development. This takes place, of course, with the backdrop of stigma and prejudice that homosexuality engenders within our society. For the African-American gay or bisexual male, the additional disrepute that his own community holds toward homosexuality makes this process more difficult to manage. A description of Troiden's (1993) four-stage model, which characterizes the path toward gay identity integration, is presented in Table 5–2. How the stages may manifest themselves differently for African-American males is discussed below.

TABLE 5–2. A Model of Sexual Identity Formation

Stage 1:	Sensitization
Stage 2:	Identity confusion
Stage 3:	Identity assumption
Stage 4:	Commitment

Stage 1: Sensitization

The first stage is characterized by feelings of difference or marginality coupled with perceptions of being different from same-sex peers. The stage is divided into early (prior to 13 years of age) and late (13–17 years) phases, and its hallmark is a sense of apartness from more conventional peers.

The literature (Bell et al. 1981, Doyle 1983, Tavris and Wade 1984) seems to indicate that most individuals during this stage are only dimly aware, if aware at all, of the nature of their sexual orientation. Before adolescence, many individuals have certain types of experiences that may later serve to identify their sexual feelings as homosexual, but at this time they do not. The types of feelings or thoughts that individuals recall experiencing during this period are alienation, feelings of inadequacy, warmth and excitement in the presence of same-sex peers, low self-esteem, and fear of rejection and ridicule. "I had a keener interest in the arts." "I couldn't stand sports, so naturally that made me different." "I was called the sissy of the family. I had been very pointedly told that I was effeminate" (Bell et al. 1981, pp. 74, 86). These statements characterize the feelings and memories many gay men have from this period of their lives. Experiences of this nature seem to produce feelings of difference in a general sense that began to crystalize into a distinct sense of sexual dissimilarity during high school, often before the age of 17. What this suggests is that it is not so much childhood experiences themselves that are important in the acquisition of gay identities, it is the meanings that are attributed to these social, emotional, and genital experiences later in life that appear to be necessary conditions for the eventual adoption of a homosexual identity (Troiden 1993).

For the gay or bisexual African-American male child or adolescent, this marginalization and feeling of difference is often heightened by the ostracism and devaluation that African-Americans encounter in American society; consequently, these young people experience multiple assaults to their self-esteem and self-confidence.

To combat the feelings experienced during the Sensitization Stage, and to prevent them from entering into conscious awareness, Coleman (1982) contends that many adolescents utilize the defense mechanisms of denial, repression, reaction formation, sublimation, and rationalization. These defenses keep individuals, their families, and society from experiencing the crisis that would occur if the issue of homosexuality were confronted directly. The consequences of this concealment can be enormously destructive. Because individuals at this stage are often not consciously aware of their same-sex feelings, they cannot describe what is wrong. They can only communicate their conflict through behavioral problems, psychosomatic illnesses, or suicide attempts.

Stage 2: Identity Confusion

The second stage is thought to begin in adolescence and is typified by the individual's beginning to reflect upon the possibility that the feelings, thoughts, or behaviors he is experiencing could be labeled gay or homosexual. This stage, characterized by a struggle to determine whether one is or is not homosexual, is a conflictual and difficult time marked by inner turmoil and confusion (Troiden 1993). The average age at which most individuals seem to be confronted by this sexual ambiguity is between 13 and 18 years (Bell et al. 1981). Troiden (1993) contends there are several factors responsible for the identity confusion experienced during this phase: (1) altered perceptions of self, (2) the experience of heterosexual and homosexual arousal and behavior, (3) an awareness of the stigma associated with homosexuality, and (4) inaccurate knowledge about homosexuals and homosexuality. Since the stigma surrounding homosexuality is so great, most gay men and lesbians struggle with this conflict in silence. A variety of different strategies are used to manage this confusion. They often include denial (disavowing the homosexual content of fantasies, feelings, and activities), avoidance (inhibiting the behaviors or interests associated with homosexuality, limiting exposure to information about homosexuality and members of the opposite sex, assuming antihomosexual postures), redefinition (attempting to interpret feelings and behaviors as temporary or unique in some manner), repair (seeking out treatment to eliminate homosexual feelings and behaviors), and acceptance (acknowledging that the feelings and behaviors may be homosexual and seeking out further information) (Cass 1979, Goode 1984, Humphreys 1972, Troiden 1977).

Denial, repair, avoidance, or redefinition may be sustained for extended periods of time. The intensity of their feelings, life circumstances, and social roles will all play a hand in determining how individuals attempt to manage the anxiety stimulated by their homosexual feelings and thoughts.

Stage Three: Identity Assumption

A sizable number of men advance to this stage during late adolescence and early adulthood. Troiden (1993) conceptualizes this stage as one in which homosexual identity becomes both a self-identity and a presented identity. Coleman (1982) and Lee (1977) write about this stage in a larger context related to the coming-out process. In essence, this stage is characterized by the individual's labeling his feelings as homosexual. The self-definition as gay, initial involvement in the gay community, and the reconfiguration of homosexuality as a positive and viable lifestyle alternative are viewed as making up the primary content of this state. Telling select others (normally other homosexual people) and affiliation with other gay men and lesbians is commonly associated with this stage of development. The quality of a person's initial contacts with homosexuals is extremely important (Cass 1979). If initial contacts are negative, further contact with homosexuals may be avoided and nonhomosexual perceptions of self will persist (Troiden 1993). African-American gay or bisexual men are often at risk for unpleasant initial contact with other homosexuals. Concern about encountering rejection and alienation from their own community leads many African-American men to seek out the white gay community for these initial contacts. Unfortunately for many, they encounter both overt and covert racism in these social settings. Loiacano (1993) describes the difficulty many African-Americans experience when they go to bars, such as being required to present three or four pieces of identification not requested of their white counterparts. Frequently they receive unfriendly service from bar staff, or encounter rejection because they do not fit white standards of beauty. At traditional gay and lesbian organizations and self-help groups their social needs and concerns are often disregarded. Consequently, the social and sexual exploration of the gay community for these individuals is often more complicated and treacherous than that of their white peers.

Positive contacts with homosexuals provide gay men with the opportunity to gain accurate and firsthand information that facilitates a reexamination of the biases and misconceptions they were socialized to adopt about homosexuality. Experienced homosexuals provide these individuals with role models, strategies to manage social stigma, and norms governing homosexual conduct (Troiden 1993).

For many there is initial relief in finally acknowledging one's gay identity; however, the pain of stigma and nonacceptance by the larger society continues to exist. To avoid this discomfort, according to Humphreys (1972), many gay people adopt one of several stigma-evasion strategies: capitulation, minstrelization, passing, and group alignment. *Capitulation* entails avoiding homosexual activity because the individual has internalized a stigmatizing view of homosexuality. *Minstrelization* involves expressing one's homosexuality along stereotypical (gender-crossed) lines. *Passing* as heterosexual is the most frequently adopted stigma-management strategy. Individuals who pass define themselves as homosexual, but conceal their sexual orientation from heterosexual family, friends, and colleagues. They often lead difficult double lives as they attempt to foster two separate social spheres (homosexual and heterosexual) that never intersect. This coping strategy is often used by African-Americans who do not want to risk being marginalized within their communities. Last, *group alignment* refers to becoming actively involved in the homosexual community. The perception of "belonging" to a world of others situated similarly eases the pain of stigma (Troiden 1993).

What is important to remember about this stage is that the homosexual feelings are often more tolerated than accepted. The oppressive fear and anxiety has been left behind, but the jacket of homosexuality is worn more with reluctance than pride.

Stage 4: Commitment

The final stage involves adopting homosexuality as a way of life. The two important aspects to keep in mind are self-acceptance and comfort with a gay identity and gay role. Commitment is viewed to have internal and external dimensions. Internal indicators include fusion of sexuality and emotionality into a significant whole (Coleman 1982, Troiden 1979, Warren 1974). Same-gender relationships are now viewed as viable and valid sources of love and romance as well as sexual satisfaction. This means that the person can enter into a relationship with someone of the same gender and be drawn to them not only sexually but also emotionally.

Another internal manifestation of a "committed" stage of development involves the perception of a gay identity as legitimate and not secondary to a heterosexual identity. Quite simply, this means that the person experiences happiness around defining himself as gay. A good way to measure this would be to ask, "If it were possible, and you could be heterosexual in the true sense of the word, would you do it?" It is theorized that the "committed" gay male would choose to remain the way he is.

External indicators include initiating and maintaining same-sex love relationships and disclosing the homosexual identity. Lee (1977) conceptualizes this coming-out process as involving disclosure of the homosexual identity to some of an expanding series of individuals ranging from the self and other homosexuals initially to heterosexual friends, family, co-workers, and employers. Few people disclose their homosexual identity to everyone in their social

sphere. Generally, as de Monteflores and Schultz (1978) postu-
late, they vary in the degree of openness, depending on personal,
social, and professional factors. The important construct here is
that the "internalized shame" present in the previous stages is well
on its way to being eradicated. Again, it is crucial to highlight that
this process may be significantly different for African-American
gay and bisexual men. The fear of being ostracized and rejected
by the African-American community (family, peers, and church),
which helps most African-Americans manage the biases and prejudice that exist in this country, makes disclosure of this nature
emotionally prohibitive. Moreover, for an African-American male to
disclose his homosexual identity at his place of work would add
another heavy "ism" to the burden of racism that often hinders his
professional advancement and promotion.

For the gay or lesbian person to develop a self-identity that
does not stigmatize homosexuality but reconceptualizes it from a
deviance to something to be exalted takes quite a while, and the
process of developing a "committed" ideology is always in a
process of becoming (Plummer 1975). Troiden (1993) suggests
that the stage of commitment may best be understood as a continuum, that is, gay people vary across time and place depending
upon the personal, social, or professional factors that impact
upon their lives. Like Atkinson and colleagues (1989), with their
formulation of ethnic-racial identity development, Troiden does
not contend that every gay person goes through the aforementioned stages in the manner he describes. He also recognizes that
socioeconomic status and level of education impact saliently upon
the process of gay identity development. Troiden's model, in
conjunction with the Atkinson and colleagues (1989) framework,
can be very helpful for the clinician who is attempting to
conceptualize the factors that have come to shape the emotional
functioning and cognitive outlook of African-American gay and
bisexual men impacted by HIV.

A Stage-Focused Treatment Model for HIV Disease

Several models presented in the psychological literature have attempted to explicate the emotional reactions individuals seem to have after receiving an HIV-positive diagnosis. The most consistent element of these models has been their incorporation of Kubler-Ross's (1969, 1987) stages of coping with terminal illness. HIV-impacted people seem to mirror Kubler-Ross's stages of Denial, Anger, Bargaining, Depression, and Acceptance. Dailey (1990) noted that the aforementioned psychological stages seem to correspond with the HIV infection cycle (see Chapter 1). Dailey has found that the initial diagnosis of seropositivity appears to correspond with a period of denial. The first HIV-related illness stimulates feelings of anger. Eventual hospitalizations induce periods of bargaining, while the realization that a terminal illness is upon them brings about depression. As death approaches, the individual ideally reaches a period of acceptance. The model proposed by Dailey is useful and provides the framework for the following discussion of the psychosocial stages of living with HIV disease, although everyone impacted by HIV will not go through the stages outlined. Moreover, for African-American gay and bisexual men, the manifestation and timing of the stages are often different from those of their heterosexual or Caucasian counterparts. These differences are highlighted below, along with recommendations for clinical intervention. Table 5–3 presents the HIV coping model.

TABLE 5–3.
A Stage-Event-Focused Model of Coping with HIV Disease

Stage 1:	Denial (HIV-positive diagnosis)
Stage 2:	Anger (first AIDS-related illness)
Stage 3:	Bargaining (multiple hospitalizations)
Stage 4:	Depression (terminal illness)
Stage 5:	Acceptance (approaching death)

Stage 1: Denial (HIV-Positive Diagnosis)

For most individuals, receiving an HIV-positive diagnosis stimulates a great deal of stress. Many people respond to situational distress with denial (Weiss 1976). According to the clinical research literature, three types of denial are commonly employed by HIV-positive persons: Primary, Secondary, and Denial without Benefit.

Primary Denial is characterized by self-deception, during which the HIV-impacted individual will discuss the realities of his situation and utilize an available support system (e.g., social service agency, physician, self-help group); these individuals seem to avoid strong affect, however, and discuss their HIV-positive status in a detached and intellectualized manner. They often make comments such as: "It doesn't bother me. I suspected that I might have been exposed to the virus." "I'm okay, there are worse things that could happen to me." "Sure, I'll come in to see you. I guess I need to learn how to take care of myself now." What seems to characterize this type of denial is the sense that the person is discussing the HIV status of someone else, not himself.

Secondary Denial is distinguished by social deception and illusion. Here the HIV-infected person is less willing to discuss his HIV status and is ambivalent or openly resistant to utilizing social service or medical resources. The emotional thrust of these individuals is to try to do everything they can not to think about or process the reality of their HIV status. Feelings of anxiety, dread, and fear threaten the individual's emotional equilibrium. To restore balance, reality is distorted and a fantasy that erases the disagreeable and unwelcome facts of the situation is created. For the HIV-impacted person this means that psychological effort is expended to create the illusion that he is HIV negative. It seems as though the person is operating from the perspective of "If I do not talk about it or think about it, then it is not real and it never happened."

Secondary Denial manifests itself in missed or tardy appointments with the medical and social service teams, inconsistence or complete noncompliance with medication protocols or behavioral interventions, and refusal to engage in dialogue with anyone (including family or significant others) about the individual's HIV-positive status. Not uncommonly, some individuals increase their alcohol or recreational drug use to sedate the feelings of anxiety and dread.

In *Denial without Benefit*, individuals do not work with a treatment team at all. These individuals, not as a result of limited financial resources or lack of knowledge about HIV, cut themselves off from anything associated with HIV. The person utilizing Secondary Denial attempts to avoid thinking or talking about HIV; an individual using Denial without Benefit tries to convince himself that he is *not* HIV positive and therefore does not have to engage in behaviors that protect his health. At times this person may take part in high-risk behaviors such as unprotected sexual intercourse, and demonstrate other signs of a lack of responsibility for his illness. The emotional thrust with Denial without Benefit is "I am not HIV positive, so I don't have to behave like I am."

Clinical Intervention Strategies

It should be pointed out that a little denial is actually efficacious if it helps to reduce the initial anxiety of the HIV-positive diagnosis (Earl et al. 1991, Mandel 1986, Price et al. 1986). Denial can be a positive reaction to counter feelings of self-blame and fear associated with HIV infection. However, over the course of the illness, denial's usefulness wears thin when active intervention is needed to address medical and psychological concerns (Sarwer and Crawford 1994).

The initial therapeutic focus for the mental health professional should be to use a crisis-intervention approach. The therapist's job is to serve as a container for the fear and anxiety associated with an HIV-positive diagnosis (Machs and Turner

1986). Therapists who are able to forge a trusting relationship with the patient and create a safe environment must be prepared for the intense affect that may be released by the patient. The therapist should attempt to reassure the patient that an HIV-positive health status does *not* automatically suggest death. The CDC reports growing numbers of individuals who have maintained good health after ten years of HIV infection (Phillips et al. 1992). Patients need to be informed of this and reminded that they may have many years of good health ahead of them. Many of their hopes, dreams, and aspirations will be realized. It becomes apparent that the therapist must not only be able to manage and mediate the patient's affective response, he/she must also be knowledgeable about HIV, its medical course, and treatments. Providing the patient with information about HIV, modes of transmission, and health maintenance and promotion is also an important task of the therapist, who at times will feel more like a health educator than a psychotherapist. If the screen of denial can be pierced, most patients will have many HIV-related questions. To be effective and to be perceived as useful, the therapist will need to be informed about HIV.

Therapists will also find themselves having to serve in the role of case manager; consequently, it will be important for the therapist to be knowledgeable about the social service and medical resources available in the community for HIV-impacted people. For therapists working with African-American gay and bisexual men, this is a very crucial component of a therapist's job. Referrals to facilities must be made carefully. Connecting these individuals with social service and medical personnel who are sensitive and informed about the cultural, social, and economic issues associated with the life experiences of these men is critical. Noncompliance and resistance to medical and social service recommendations among African-American gay and bisexual men can often result from a lack of trust that these individuals have toward their treatment team; therefore, if mental health professionals can make an *informed* referral to someone they know will relate effectively with their patient, the likelihood of a successful outcome is greatly enhanced. It should be kept in mind that if a patient has been able to form a relationship with his therapist, then a certain degree of trust has been established. If the patient is directed to someone the therapist believes in, then the patient may approach that individual or facility with less trepidation.

Most African-American gay and bisexual men discover their HIV-positive status during what turns out to be their first AIDS-related illness. Few of these individuals will seek out HIV antibody testing if their health status is good; consequently, this group of Americans often experiences the double blow of learning they are not only HIV positive, but also carry a diagnosis of AIDS. As a result, most mental health professionals are likely to encounter African-American gay and bisexual men who are experiencing emotional reactions associated with Stage 2: Anger.

Stage 2: Anger (First AIDS-Related Illness)

The first AIDS-related illness often moves the patient from denial to an anger style of coping (Dailey 1990); in the case of African-American gay and bisexual men, however, this is often the first psychological stage of coping they encounter. The target of the anger may be many things. Due to the stigmatizing nature of HIV disease, many persons with AIDS become socially isolated, and the target of the anger is often directed at those agents they perceive stigmatize them and hold them in disdain (Sarwer and Crawford 1994). The anger is often directed at the individual who infected him, people who are HIV negative, or members of his social support system or medical treatment team. It seems that the anger is a manifestation of feeling frustrated and exasperated by being ill and no longer "normal" like everyone else. It is not uncommon for the HIV-impacted person to isolate himself during this time. It appears this occurs when the anger becomes internalized and clients experience feelings of self-hatred. Coates and colleagues (1984) report that gay HIV-impacted patients may experience this hatred in the form of self-condemnation and guilt. The affective responses to HIV disease can cause some gay and bisexual men to question themselves about previously resolved aspects of their identity that had been pushed out of conscious awareness. It would be helpful for the therapist to keep in mind the model of gay identity development discussed previously. It is not uncommon for the chinks in the gay identity armor to become magnified by the feelings of stigmatization that HIV carries in our society. For the African-American gay or bisexual male this may also stimulate threats to the self related to the self-hating, conformity stage of racial identity development. The public face of AIDS is changing in the United States from the affluent, Caucasian gay male to the injection-drug-using, lower-income, ethnic-racial minority generally held in contempt by society. To recognize that the citizenry largely associates you with this group can be a significant assault to one's self-esteem.

Clinical Intervention Strategies

The therapeutic tasks of the mental health professional for individuals in this stage of coping are to provide social support and a safe place for the patient to express his anger and frustration. The use of social support and psychotherapy groups has been found effective in helping these individuals manage their anger. The groups help to address the problem of social isolation and also give patients an environment in which it is safe to express sometimes overwhelming and dangerous emotions. The expression of anger is important, for it provides the patient with the opportunity to confront and address the feelings that are at the core of the anger and develop a sense of control over them.

While support groups can be very useful at this time, the literature suggests that group cohesion and therapeutic focus are extremely important factors that must be monitored and maintained closely. To increase cohesiveness, Spector and Conklin

(1987) suggest forming groups on the basis of health, such that members share similar health issues and feelings of fear and denial. In addition to providing a safe outlet for the expression of feelings, group work should also incorporate a cognitive-behavioral or psychoeducational focus. Group participants should be able to learn from their fellow group members or group facilitator how to cope effectively with threatening feelings (e.g., fear, anger, isolation, recrimination) or situations (accessing medical or social service resources; disclosing HIV status to family, friends, co-workers, employer). What appears to be most iatrogenic are groups or individual psychotherapy sessions that allow the patient to focus only on negative affect and events that are out of his control.

Pincu (1989) and Quadland and Shattis (1987) believe that many HIV-positive men use sex to combat feelings of loneliness and to decrease the anxiety of socializing. Group or individual therapy that examines culturally defined gender roles and attitudes toward sex have been shown to be quite effective in reducing risk-taking sexual behaviors (Kelly et al. 1993, Price et al. 1986). Again, using a cognitive-behavioral therapeutic framework that initially explores the feelings associated with compulsive sexual behavior, followed by an examination of the actual behaviors, thoughts, and cues that lead to unsafe sexual practices, has been found to be effective in disrupting the behavioral cycle and allowing these men to develop a greater sense of self-efficacy.

For African-American gay and bisexual men, the constellation of the group is extremely important to their therapeutic effectiveness. Variables of socioeconomic status, sexual orientation, and race need to be taken into consideration as much as possible. Assessing the stage of racial and sexual identity development of the individual before a referral is made or an individual is assigned to a group is crucial. For example, assigning an HIV-infected African-American bisexual male who is in the Conformity (Racial) and Identity Confusion (Sexual) stages of development to a group that primarily consists of Caucasian gay men who are in the Commitment stage of their gay identity would probably be a suboptimal assignment. For these groups to work effectively, trust, shared experiences, and emotional safety must be present. It is the therapist's job to create these environments.

Stage 3: Bargaining (Multiple Hospitalizations)

The onset of HIV-associated medical complications and illnesses that lead to multiple hospitalizations appears to bring about a brief period of bargaining for people living with the disease. According to Kubler-Ross (1969), bargaining may involve specific sacrifices or attempts to be a better person in general, with the reward of a longer life or days without pain or discomfort. Perhaps for the first time since the initial diagnosis, the patient now begins to realize that his health and life are challenged by HIV. Fears of death and illness become salient (Walker 1991).

The primary feeling that seems to accompany the Bargaining Stage is guilt (Coates et al. 1984, Walker 1991). Guilt that is directed at one's sexual orientation, sexual practices, or substance abuse history is common during this stage. It is also not unusual for patients to express culpability for not meeting parental expectations or outliving friends who died of AIDS.

Clinical Intervention Strategies

Supportive psychotherapy and social support groups are useful during this stage. Moreover, mental health professionals may want to consider recommending or supporting the patient's involvement with religion or spirituality. Many people turn to religion as they confront the reality of death. It would be useful for the therapist to explore with the client the role religion or spirituality has played in their lives and to what degree it might be helpful to them at this time. Walker (1991) and Winiarski (1991) have found that religion has assisted many HIV-impacted individuals in dealing with feelings of guilt, giving them a sense of belonging and community.

For many African-American patients living with AIDS, the practice of religion and spiritualism becomes a primary coping strategy. Individuals who may not have expressed strong religious or spiritual beliefs in the past may now articulate a need to "reconnect" or "get their house in order with the Lord." As mentioned earlier, the black church has been a sustaining element in the social history of African-Americans. When under stress or in crisis, faith and the community of the church have been constants that African-Americans have relied upon. Therapists need to appreciate the cultural context of religion for their African-American patients, and be willing to work with them as they identify a comfortable and useful role for the church in their lives.

It should be pointed out that mental health professionals can also assist their clients in this stage by encouraging them to engage in an active living style of coping with HIV/AIDS. Assisting the client in developing and maintaining a health program of nutrition, exercise, rest, and abstinence from recreational drugs and alcohol is also a necessary therapeutic task (Kelly 1989).

Stage 4: Depression (Terminal Illness)

When bargaining fails, individuals coping with a terminal illness enter a period of depression. The realization that the medical condition the person is battling against is one he cannot win often leads to feelings of helplessness, sadness, and defeat. Much of the depression appears to be stimulated by the experiences of many losses, such as the loss of self-esteem, independence, mobility, physical appearance, sexual relationships, and social contacts (Morin et al. 1984, Price et al. 1986, Quadland and Shattis 1987). An individual at this stage is confronted with the stark reality that his life has changed; regardless of what he does, he cannot reclaim it, and the eventuality of his death has become tangible. Concomitant with the emotional dysphoria of these realizations, HIV-impacted people at this stage are also confronted with specific physical symptomatology and loss of functioning. Several researchers (Coates et al. 1984, Kiecolt-Glaser and Glaser 1988) have recognized that the stress and anxiety accompanying this stage may also have an adverse effect upon the immune system functioning of late-stage HIV-infected individuals, which further compromises the health status of the patient. The combination of feelings of depression and anxiety, along with physical deterioration and pain, often leads to the development of suicidal ideation at this stage of coping with HIV disease. Not only is suicidal ideation common in persons living with AIDS, but these persons also have higher suicide rates than the general population (Frierson and Lippmann 1987, Kizer et al. 1988, Marzuk et al. 1988). Moreover, Frierson and Lippmann note that when patients experience depression at this stage without the presence of a viable support system, the development of suicidal ideation is greatly enhanced.

Clinical Intervention Strategies

Mental health professionals working with patients at this stage of HIV illness should conduct a thorough assessment of the patient's affective experience, paying particular attention to the possibility of suicidal ideation. Therapists are advised to talk openly about suicide with their clients, and carefully assess thoughts, intentions, plans, and actual attempts (Sarwer and Crawford 1994). If depression and suicidality are present, clinical intervention should be swift and pointed. Based on the work of Coates and McKusick (1987) and Kelly and colleagues (1993), two primary tasks should be on the mental health professional's agenda. First, in either an individual or group therapy context, the professional should attempt to create a safe and supportive environment that will allow the client to vent the emotions associated with the many losses he has endured, his fears or anxieties associated with death, and other feelings or thoughts related to living with AIDS. Second, intervention should focus on assisting the patient in managing the stress associated with HIV disease at this stage of the illness. Cognitive behavioral approaches that provide skills to manage and reduce stress appear to be essential in this process. These approaches seem to assist patients in decreasing maladaptive coping strategies (i.e., recreational drug use, high-risk sexual activity, medication noncompliance, and poor self-care functions), while the social support approach is effective in reducing psychological symptomatology and emotional dysphoria (Sarwer and Crawford 1994). In summary, therapists not only need to provide the client with empathy and understanding, they must also empower the patient with skills to directly combat the stress he encounters in his life.

Depressive symptomatology should not be viewed as inevitable or unmanageable in the person living with AIDS. Mental health professionals must understand that the prevention or effective treatment of depression can extend life and elevate health status (Maj 1990). If behavioral strategies do not produce timely or significantly beneficial results, therapists may want to consider augmenting treatment with antidepressant or other psychotropic medications (Sarwer and Crawford 1994).

In addition to having to manage depressive symptomatology, many patients are also confronted with the reality that they can no longer hide the nature of their illness or sexual orientation. For some men this may lead to another coming-out process. The person living with AIDS may be challenged to divulge his HIV/AIDS diagnosis to his co-workers, employer, friends, and family. Many of the same anxieties and fears discussed in reference to the coming-out process related to sexual identity arise in this context (Nichols 1986). Shaw (1992) writes that revealing one's AIDS diagnosis can be a particularly turbulent and upsetting experience for these individuals. Not only do these men experience feelings of anxiety related to potential rejection or derision, having to disclose this information to others shatters the last vestiges of denial the person has related to his ability to overcome HIV.

For African-American gay and bisexual men living with AIDS, this can be an even more disturbing experience. As previously discussed, many of these men do not disclose their sexual orientation to their families. So they now find themselves having to tell their families not only that they have AIDS, but that they are also gay or bisexual. Fear of familial rejection and feelings of disappointment and recrimination often surface during this time. Mental health professionals may be of assistance at this time by providing support, reminding patients of the networks they have in place that they can rely upon, and discussing how they will respond if they receive positive or negative reactions to their disclosures. Developing coping plans for these potential reactions are extremely important. If the reaction is poor, a coping plan could be, "I will go home and meditate or pray for fifteen minutes and then call my friend _____ , or if I am really upset, I will call my therapist or another member of my medical team to talk things out." The primary point here is that patients need to have a sense that they will know what to do if negative feelings arise. It would not be unusual, and is often indicated, for the mental health professional to conduct family therapy sessions with the patient and his family to assist in the disclosure and processing of subsequent feelings and reactions. If a therapist can assist the process and increase the potential for a positive outcome, the therapeutic impact on the patient can be immense. Mandel (1986) reports the "coming out" with AIDS may actually increase one's social support network if it is done within an accepting community. If the community is not accepting, however, in fact is rejecting, the therapist's task is to provide a sense of connectedness with the patient and help him in strengthening and/or developing relationships with members of his nonbiological family and treatment team.

Mental health professionals must always work closely with their client's medical team, keeping abreast of the patient's medical status and treatment protocol (Walker 1991). Therapists should also be sensitive to the manifestation of AIDS-related dementias. Although symptoms may have appeared at earlier stages of the illness, they are often more pronounced at this juncture. Organic impairment at this time may begin to interfere with the ability of the patient to cognitively process information, which could limit the effectiveness of psychotherapeutic intervention (Sarwer and Crawford 1994).

Stage 5: Acceptance (Approaching Death)

As death approaches, patients often become more accepting of the disease and themselves. For many, death no longer stimulates intense fear or anxiety. A sense of calm and acceptance often develops at this stage; a more stable sense of self that arises out of rational reason seems to moderate the anxiety and fear that was present in the previous state (Nichols 1985). Achieving this state of grace allows individuals to make their last wishes known, heal old wounds, and begin to say good-bye (Walker 1991).

Clinical Intervention Strategies

Much of the work of the therapist in this stage is of an existential or humanistic level. Assisting the client in clarifying the meaning they have extracted out of their existence is a common task at this point. Borden (1989) recommends conducting a "life review" with the patient that will allow him to regain a cohesive sense of self (Who are you? What type of person did you create?), a carrying out of social and psychological tasks (What did you achieve in this life that you are most proud of? How did you overcome the barriers that got in your way? What did you learn about other people and yourself as you got older? What do you want the people that love you the most to remember about you?), and a final review of life (What was the happiest moment in your childhood, teenage years, adulthood? What is life about?). An examination of life in this manner will aid the patient in reaching peace with himself and the life he has led. For African-American gay or bisexual clients, this may involve a resolution of sexual and/or racial identity conflicts. Spirituality and religion also become prominent themes as death approaches. Supporting the patient's beliefs and religious practices is a very important task for the therapist at this juncture.

It is also important for mental health professionals to say good-bye to their clients, let them know they will be missed, and that their lives have been enriched by their work together. When the patient dies, if the therapist has formed professional relationships with the support system of the patient and unresolved feelings remain, the therapist should also remain available to them (Parkes 1983).

CONCLUSION

It is hoped that this presentation of the social, cultural, and intrapersonal factors that affect HIV-impacted African-American gay and bisexual men will assist mental health professionals who encounter these men in their professional work. It is important to keep in mind that the models discussed here should serve only as frameworks, and that every patient should be treated as an individual. It is an idiographic approach that distinguishes a culturally sensitive therapeutic method.

REFERENCES

Akbar, N. (1984). Afrocentric social sciences for human liberation. *Journal of Black Studies* 14:395–414.

Atkinson, D., Morten, G., and Sue, D. (1989). A minority identity development model. In *Counseling American Minorities: A Cross Cultural Perspective*, ed. Atkinson et al. (pp. 35–47). Dubuque: Wm. C. Brown.

Bell, A., Weinberg, M., and Hammersmith, S. (1981). *Sexual Preference: Its Development in Men and Women*. Bloomington: Indiana University Press.

Borden, W. (1989). Life review as a therapeutic frame in the treatment of young adults with AIDS. *Health and Social Work* 36: 253–258.

Carney, C. G., and Kahn, K. B. (1984). Building competencies for effective cross-cultural counseling: a developmental view. *The Counseling Psychologist* 12:111–119.

Cass, V. C. (1979). Homosexual identity formation: a theoretical model. *Journal of Homosexuality* 4:219–235.

——— (1984). Homosexuality identity formation: testing a theoretical model. *Journal of Sex Research* 20:143–167.

Centers for Disease Control and Prevention (CDC). (1995). *HIV/AIDS Surveillance Report* 6(1):8–18.

Chimezie, A. (1985). Black bi-culturality. *Western Journal of Black Studies* 9:224–235.

Coates, T. J., Temoshok, L., and Mandel, J. (1984). Psychosocial research is essential to understanding and treating AIDS. *American Psychologist* 39:1309–1314.

Coates, T. J., and McKusick, L. (1987). *The efficacy of stress management in reducing high-risk behavior and improving immune functioning in HIV antibody positive men*. Paper presented at the Third International Conference on AIDS.

Coleman, E. (1982). Developmental stages of the coming out process. In *Homosexuality: Social, Psychological and Biological issues*, ed. W. Paul, J. D. Weinrich, J. C. Gonsiorek, and M. E. Hotvedt, pp. 149–158. Beverly Hills, CA: Sage Publications.

Cross, W. E. (1971). The negro to black conversion experience. *Black World* 20:13–27.

Dailey, L. (1990). Therapy with inner city AIDS clients. In *New Directions for Mental Health Sciences*, ed. T. A. Kupers. New York: Jossey-Bass.

Dalton, H. (1989). AIDS in blackface. *Daedalus* 118:205–227.

de Monteflores, C., and Schultz, S. (1978). Coming out: similarities and differences for lesbians and gay men. *Journal of Social Issues* 34:59–72.

Doyle, J. (1983). *The male experience*. Dubuque: Wm. C. Brown.

Earl, W. L., Martindale, C. J., and Cohn, D. (1991). Adjustment: denial in the styles of coping with HIV infection. *Omega* 24:35–47.

Frierson, R. L., and Lippmann, S. (1987). Psychological implications of AIDS. *American Family Physician* 35:109–116.

Goode, E. (1984). *Deviant Behavior*, 2nd ed. Englewood Cliffs, NJ: Prentice-Hall.

Greene, B. (1994). Ethnic minority lesbians and gay men: mental health and treatment issues. *Journal of Consulting and Clinical Psychology* 62:243–251.

Helms, J. E. (1993). *Black and white racial identity*. Westport, CT: Praeger.

Herek, G., and Capitanio, J. (1995). Black heterosexuals' attitudes towards lesbians and gay men in the United States. *Journal of Sex Research* 32(2):95–105.

Humphreys, L. (1972). *Out of the Closets: The Sociology of Homosexual Liberation*. Englewood Cliffs, NJ: Prentice-Hall.

Jones, J., and Block, C. (1984). Black cultural perspectives. *The Clinical Psychologist* 58–62.

Kelly, J. A. (1989). Helping patients cope with AIDS and HIV conditions. *Comprehensive Therapy* 15:56–62.

Kelly, J. A., Murphy, D., Bahr, R., Kalichman, S., et al. (1993). Outcome of cognitive-behavioral and support group brief therapies for depressed persons diagnosed with HIV infection. *American Journal of Psychiatry* 150(11):1679–1686.

Kiecolt-Glaser, J. K., and Glaser, R. (1988). Psychological influences on immunity. *American Psychologist* 43:892–898.

Kizer, K., Green, M., Perkins, C., Doebbert, G., et al. (1988). AIDS and suicide in California. *Journal of the American Medical Association* 260:1181.

Kubler-Ross, E. (1969). *On Death and Dying*. New York: Macmillan.

———— (1987). *AIDS: The Ultimate Challenge*. New York: Macmillan.

Lee, J. A. (1977). Going public: a study in the sociology of homosexual liberation. *Journal of Homosexuality* 3:49–78.

Loiacano, D. (1993). Gay identity issues among black Americans: racism, homophobia, and the need for validation. In *Psychological Perspectives on Lesbian and Gay Male Experiences*, ed. L. Garnets and D. Kimmel, pp. 364–375. New York: Columbia University Press.

Machs, J., and Turner, D. (1986). Mental health issues of persons with AIDS. In *What to Do about AIDS*, ed. L. McKusick, pp. 111–124. Berkeley: University of California Press.

Maj, M. (1990). Psychiatric aspects of HIV-1 infection and AIDS. *Psychological Medicine* 20:547–563.

Mandel, J. S. (1986). Psychosocial challenges of AIDS and ARC: clinical and research findings. In *What to Do about AIDS*, ed. L. McKusick, pp. 75–86. Berkeley: University of California Press.

Marzuk, P. M., Tierney, H., Tardiff, K., Gross, E., et al. (1988). Increased risk of suicide in persons with AIDS. *Journal of the American Medical Association* 259:133–1337.

Mays, V. M. (1989). AIDS prevention in black populations: methods of a safer kind. In *Primary Prevention of AIDS: Psychological Approaches*, ed. V. M. Mays, G. W. Albee, and S. F. Schneider, pp. 264–279. Thousand Oaks, CA: Sage.

Michael, R., Gagnon, J., Laumann, E., and Kolata, G. (1994). *Sex in America: A Definitive Study*. Boston: Little, Brown.

Morin, S. F., Charles, K., and Maylon, A. (1984). The psychological impact of AIDS on gay men. *American Psychologist* 39:1288–1293.

Myers, L., Speight, S., Highlen, P., Cox, C., et al. (1991). Identity development and worldview: toward an optimal conceptualization. *Journal of Counseling and Development* 70:54–63.

Nichols, S. (1985). Psychosocial reactions of people with AIDS. *Annals of Internal Medicine* 103:765–767.

———— (1986). Psychotherapy and AIDS. In *Contemporary Perspectives on Psychotherapy with Lesbians and Gay Men*, ed. T. S. Stein and C. J. Cohen, pp. 209–239. New York: Plenum.

Parham, T. A. (1981). The influence of black students' racial identity on preference for counselor's race. *Journal of Counseling Psychology* 28:250–257.

Parkes, C. M. (1983). *Recovery from Bereavement*. New York: Basic Books.

Paterson, L. (1983). At Ebenezer baptist church. In *Black Men/White Men: A Gay Anthology*, ed. M. J. Smith, pp. 163–167. San Francisco: Gay Sunshine.

Peterson, J. L. (1992). Black men and their same sex desires and behaviors. In *Gay Culture in America: Essays from the Field*, ed. G. Herdt, pp. 147–164. Boston: Beacon.

Phillips, A., Elford, J., Sabin, C., Bofill, M., et al. (1992). Immunodeficiency and the risk of death in HIV infection. *Journal of the American Medical Association* 18:2662–2666.

Pincu, L. (1989). Sexual compulsivity in gay men: controversy and treatment. *Journal of Counseling and Development* 68:63–66.

Plummer, K. (1975). *Sexual Stigma: An Interactionist Account*. London: Routledge/Kegan Paul.

Ponse, B. (1978). *Identities in the Lesbian World: The Social Construction of Self*. Westport, CT: Greenwood.

Ponterotto, J. G. (1988). Racial consciousness development among white counselor trainees. *Journal of Multicultural Counseling and Development* 16:146–156.

Price, R. E., Omizo, M. M., and Hammett, V. (1986). Counseling clients with AIDS. *Journal of Counseling and Development* 65:96–97.

Quadland, M., and Shattis, W. (1987). AIDS, sexuality and sexual control. *Journal of Homosexuality* 14:277–298.

Ruiz, R. A., and Padilla, A. M. (1977). Counseling Latinos. *Personal and Guidance Journal* 55:401–408.

Sarwer, D., and Crawford, I. (1994). Therapeutic considerations for work with persons with HIV disease. *Psychotherapy* 31:262–269.

Schäfer, S. (1976). Sexual and social problems among lesbians. *Journal of Sexual Research* 12:50–69.

Shaw, S. (1992). Psychotherapy of the HIV-positive patient and family: an integrated approach. In *Living and Dying with AIDS*, ed. P. I. Ahmed, pp. 87–102. New York: Plenum.

Spector, I., and Conklin, R. (1987). AIDS group psychotherapy. *International Journal of Group Psychotherapy* 37:433–439.

Sue, D. W., and Sue, D. (1990). *Counseling the Culturally Different: Theory and Practice.* New York: Wiley.

Tavris, C., and Wade, C. (1984). *The Longest War: Sex Differences in Perspective.* New York: Harcourt Brace Jovanovich.

Thomas, S., and Quinn, S. (1991). The Tuskegee syphilis study, 1932 to 1972: implications for HIV education and AIDS risk education programs in the black community. *American Journal of Public Health* 81(11):1498–1505.

Troiden, R. R. (1977). Becoming homosexual: a model of gay identity acquisition. *Psychiatry* 42:362–373.

——— (1979). *Becoming homosexual: research on acquiring a gay identity.* Unpublished doctoral dissertation, State University of New York at Stony Brook.

——— (1993). The formation of homosexual identities. In *Psychological Perspectives on Lesbian and Gay Male Experiences*, ed. L. Garnets and D. Kimmel, pp. 191–217. New York: Columbia University Press.

Walker, G. (1991). *In the Midst of Winter: Systemic Therapy with Families, Couples, and Individuals with AIDS Infections.* New York: Norton.

Warren, C. (1974). *Identity and Community in the Gay World.* New York: Wiley.

Weinberg, T. S. (1978). On doing and being gay: sexual behavior and homosexual male self-identity. *Journal of Homosexuality* 4:143–156.

Weiss, R. S. (1976). Transition states and other stressful situations: their nature and programs for their management. In *Support Systems and Mutual Help*, ed. G. Caplan and M. Killilea. New York: Grune and Stratton.

Winiarski, M. (1991). *AIDS-Related Psychotherapy*. New York: Pergamon.

6

Treating the HIV-Impacted Hispanic Male Client

TOMAS SOTO

INTRODUCTION

The HIV/AIDS epidemic continues to disproportionately impact the Hispanic community. Unfortunately, knowledge regarding effective prevention strategies and treatment interventions for this community is not developing at the same pace as the epidemic or the growth of the Hispanic population in the United States. This fastest-growing minority group is expected to become the largest minority group in the country by the year 2010. While research has begun to examine cultural variables associated with HIV/AIDS prevention for the Hispanic population (Marin 1989), with few exceptions, articles have not focused on the mental health treatment of HIV-infected Hispanics (Bing and Soto 1991, Carballo-Dieguez 1989).

This chapter aims to increase the understanding of how cultural considerations (gender role dichotomization, ethnic identity formation, familialism, religion) and individual variables (language, sexual identity development, immigration status, childhood sexual abuse, maladaptive coping strategies) impact treatment interventions for the Hispanic male client throughout the stages of HIV progression. Treatment issues relevant to Hispanic women and children are discussed in Chapter 7.

EPIDEMIOLOGY

The HIV/AIDS epidemic is disproportionately represented in the Hispanic community. According to the 1990 census, Hispanics represent roughly 9 percent of the country's population yet constitute 17 percent of the reported adult and adolescent AIDS cases (CDC 1995). The AIDS incidence rate for all Hispanics has increased dramatically (13.5 percent from 1989 to 1995). In 1995 the CDC reported that the AIDS incidence rate was two and a half times higher for Hispanic men than for non-Hispanic white men. Cumulatively, the CDC (1995) reports 68,051 cases of AIDS among Hispanic/Latino men through June 1995. Of that total, 45 percent report being exposed to the virus through male-to-male sexual contact. Thirty-eight percent are exposed through injection drug use; an additional 7 percent report both male sexual contact and injection drug use. Heterosexual transmission of HIV accounts for 4 percent of the cases in this population; blood transfusions for 1 percent. For 6 percent of reported Hispanic male cases the transmission source is unknown or yet to be determined.

What we have learned from these numbers is that Hispanic men are being infected at alarmingly high rates and are exposed to the virus predominantly through male-to-male sexual contact, injection drug use, and heterosexual contact. The mode of transmission often yields important clinical data for understanding the experience of the HIV-infected Hispanic male. The growing number of Hispanic men contracting the virus signifies a need for psychological services and support for these individuals.

MODE OF TRANSMISSION

Transmission via male-to-male sexual contact can take a variety of different forms. Given this reality, the term *men who have sex with men* has replaced the terms *gay* or *bisexual* when collectively describing same-sex sexual behavior. Carballo-Dieguez and Dolezal (1994a), in a study of Puerto Rican men, note four contrasting types of men who have sex with men: (1) heterosexual men who have sex with men, (2) bisexual men who have sex with men, (3) gay men who have sex with men, and (4) transvestites (drag queens). They note similarities within the groups in relation to age and members infected, yet found significant differences between groups in socio-economic status, attitudes, and behaviors.

Specifically, heterosexual men who had sex with men viewed themselves no differently than exclusively heterosexual Hispanic men and they consistently externalized responsibility for their sexual acts with men, attributing the incidents to situational factors. From a psychological perspective, one can speculate that this subpopulation of men has a strong need to avoid internalizing same-sex attraction. As internalizing this behavior would create psychological conflict, dissociation becomes a primary defense. Bisexual men who have sex with men reported relations with both men and women, either simultaneously or sequentially, and showed more versatility in their sexual practices with men. This seems to suggest a slightly higher level of comfort with male-to-male sexual behavior. Gay men who had sex with men had the highest income and educational level of the four groups and the lowest levels of homophobia. Finally, the transvestite subpopulation, which very much viewed themselves as female both in mannerism and dress, were the most disenfranchised of the four groups. They had lower levels of education and income, with many supporting themselves through commercial sex. This seminal research provides a foundation from which to better understand the psychological and behavioral variables that shape some aspects of Hispanic male sexuality. Sensitivity and consideration should be given to how Hispanic men who have sex with men choose to manage their sexual behaviors and thoughts.

In addition to male-to-male transmission of the virus, a significant percentage of Hispanic men contract the virus through injection drug use. This subpopulation of Hispanic men shares cultural and gender-related similarities with other HIV-impacted Hispanic men. The differences lie in the development of a separate substance-abuse problem that is superimposed on the aforementioned challenges. (Specific discussion of the dynamics of substance abuse and HIV are discussed in Chapter 8.) Suffice it to say, the clinician working with the substance-abusing Hispanic male has additional problematic areas to assess that will make treatment planning more complex.

The previous discussion highlights the variability that exists among Hispanic men who contract HIV. The contribution of Hispanic male gender role socialization, sexual and racial/ethnic identity formation, and overarching context of Hispanic culture: all play significant parts in the emotional reactions Hispanic men experience when confronted by HIV disease. These salient factors are discussed below in greater detail.

Cultural Consideration

Within Hispanic culture, as with any culture, there are primary, overarching cultural constructs that impact psychological development. It is important to have a clear understanding of these overriding cultural constructs and their impact on individuals prior to delivering mental health services to Hispanic men. Hispanic identity development is shaped by various factors (family, geographic region, religion, and many others). A discussion of all the factors impacting Hispanic male identity development is beyond the scope of this chapter. Yet certain factors, specifically gender role socialization, level of acculturation, familialism, and religion, seem to be of great importance in relation to the management of HIV infection. Emphasis is given here to the impact of Hispanic culture on these variables in the hope that a keen understanding of the interface of these variables can aid in the assessment and treatment of HIV-impacted Hispanic men.

Male Gender Identity

It is not uncommon for young Hispanic boys to be told "tu tienes que ser un hombre macho" (you need to become a macho man). These messages are given early and become internalized as they begin to grow up to become men. What does it mean to be "macho"? Although hispanic masculinity has not been studied exclusively, there is a growing body of literature beginning to show the negative psychological consequences associated with adherence to rigid male gender role adherence (Eisler and Skidmore 1987, Flannery 1978). Specifically, men are socialized to adopt a rather firm set of expectations regarding the management and expression of their feelings. Levinson (1978) interviewed a group of men in an attempt to understand what they associated with being male and found the following characteristics:

- Having power, exercising control, and being recognized as a leader
- Possessing strength, toughness, and stamina, and an ability to endure bodily stress
- Possessing logical and analytical thought and intellectual competency
- Being a high achiever and having a need to be successful

While these characteristics are generalized to most men in this country, how applicable are they to Hispanic men? Specifically, to what extent does male gender role socialization impact development and how does it impact psychological functioning?

It has been shown that there is a sharp dichotomization of gender roles within Hispanic culture (Carrier 1985). We also know that machismo is often viewed as "hypermasculinity" that emphasizes emotional restrictiveness, power, and control. Appreciation of the psychological construct of machismo is a necessary prerequisite in providing effective treatment to Hispanic men. Machismo literally means maleness and virility. The culture expects the male to be the provider, the one responsible for the welfare and honor of the family, and a great deal of power and authority is given to the male. Within the sociocultural context of the Hispanic community machismo is often associated only with sexual freedom, emotional detachment, dominance over women, and excessive alcohol use. Unfortunately, these extreme behaviors are frequently internalized to varying degrees among most Hispanic men. Existing within this rigid sex role, with few, if any, emotional outlets, can cause impairment in psychological and physical functioning. In fact, Pennebaker (1992) believes that chronic repression of negative affect may be related to negative health consequences. It is the adherence to the macho image that appears to keep many Hispanic men from accessing traditional mental health services. Seeking help from others for one's emotional problems is antithetical to being a "man." Many men, regardless of ethnicity, may be more comfortable seeking medical attention before or instead of psychological counseling (Sutkin and Good 1987). For this reason mental health professionals must attempt to build solid working relationships with medical practitioners, particularly when working with individuals impacted by HIV. It is important to make sure that reported physical ailments are ruled out medically before psychological causes for physical distress are explored. In addition to psychosomatic symptomology, Hispanic men may develop maladaptive coping strategies (covered later in this chapter) such as substance abuse.

When Hispanic men contract HIV, they are faced by what the author terms *loss of machismo*. The very attributes that define what a Hispanic male should be or do are slowly taken away. The sexual freedom that symbolized virility is replaced with reminders of the virus or of being different. Redevelopment of a healthy sexual drive is often challenging. The power and strength associated with being macho are replaced with multiple illnesses and fatigue. The ability to be a provider for the family is often compromised if the Hispanic male must go on disability or is no longer able to work. Finally, family honor may suffer considerably if the family or client believes he has disgraced the family. The cumulative effects of this slow dismantling of the client's masculinity, once a source of pride and self-worth, can be emotionally overwhelming. A clinician must be empathetic to these losses, real or perceived, and help the client redefine his masculinity or machismo. In order to do this, a supportive therapeutic relationship must be formed. Some latitude may need to be given to treatment structure, given that seeking therapy itself can be experienced by some as a compromise to their masculinity. Traditional treatment approaches (e.g., weekly fifty-minute sessions) may need to be modified while the client adjusts to seeking treatment. These adjustments may include episodic contact as opposed to weekly sessions, or more personalism (a valued social construct for Hispanics) during the various phases of treatment. Although no empirical research has been conducted examining levels of machismo and potential psychological distress, the clinical experience of this author supports the contention that the degree to which a Hispanic male adheres to the macho gender role may dictate the degree of psychological stress experienced. An effective treatment intervention used by this author is to work with the client in redefining machismo. This includes reclaiming aspects of the word's earlier definition, which include chivalrous behavior, charitability, and courage. Reframing the concept of machismo can be a tool in helping the client confront his HIV/AIDS with courage and dignity.

Ethnic Identity Development

While all men struggle with male gender role socialization, Hispanic men in the United States have an additional element to integrate. This element/process involves development of a healthy ethnic identity. This process, Ethnic Identity Formation, occurs simultaneously to one's developing male identity.

Ethnic Identity Formation is a process in which one tries to answer a basic question: "Who am I?" Ethnicity plays a powerful role in shaping one's view of self in relation to one's ethnic group of origin and self-identification. Bernal and Knight (1993) define ethnic identity as a set of "self ideas" (i.e., beliefs about oneself and one's ethnicity) about one's own ethnic group membership. These authors perceive this process to have many dimensions.

One dimension is self-identification, which can be defined as the ethnic terms or labels that people use to identify themselves and the meanings associated with these labels. A second dimension is an individual's knowledge about his ethnic culture; thus knowing oneself requires a knowledge of cultural history. The last dimension that Bernal and Knight (1993) discuss is the feelings, preferences, and values that an individual may have about his or her ethnic group. He or she may embrace, reject, or have neutral feelings and preferences about family, companions, and cultural values. It is important to understand these dimensions since they often impact upon how ethnic clients approach services, particularly mental health services. If a Hispanic male client embraces his ethnic identity, he may view mental health practitioners as treating only severely disturbed people and thus be reticent to seek mental health care or use other more culturally based sources of support such as the clergy. Conversely, if a client rejects his ethnic identity he may embrace Western traditions and view them as superior to those of his own culture and may enter treatment expecting a "cure" or immediate symptom relief. In either case, an assessment of the client's level of familiarity with counseling and psychotherapy is strongly recommended.

How do these dimensions of ethnic self-ideas develop in an individual? Atkinson and colleagues (1989) developed a model of five stages of development that oppressed people experience as they struggle to understand themselves in terms of their own culture, the dominant culture, other minorities, and the oppressive relationship the dominant culture has with them.

As outlined in Chapter 5, Atkinson and colleagues (1989) view oppressed individuals struggling with the integration and acceptance of their own culture and the dominant culture. In Stage 1, Conformity, an individual can be seen as almost idealizing many aspects of the dominant culture while simultaneously devaluing his own ethnic origin. A clear preference for the dominant culture is evident. This is often seen among recent immigrants as well as individuals who have left their country due to some sort of hardship. To illustrate how this information has applicability for mental health work, a description of an incident that occurred at a public medical clinic is presented below.

A gay-identified Hispanic male client referred to a mental health clinician reported dissatisfaction with his medical treatment provider, who happened to be African-American. The client had been living in a predominantly Anglo gay community on the north side of Chicago and rarely went to Hispanic neighborhoods. His previous private insurance had paid for the services of a Caucasian medical provider. When asked about his dissatisfaction with his current medical provider, he was rather vague, yet insisted on requesting an Anglo physician. When asked what he would like in a medical provider he said he wanted a doctor like his old doctor whom he trusted. While not minimizing the aspect of familiarity and trust, it seemed clear that the doctor's race was an issue. In this situation the client may be in the Conformity Stage in relation to his ethnic identity development: believing an Anglo physician to be more trustworthy, thus buying into a stereotypical belief that an Anglo doctor is more competently trained. This example demonstrates how consideration should be given to making appropriate referrals that are congruent with the context of the client. Although one would not want to endorse stereotypical beliefs that a client may hold, goodness of fit in therapeutic situations should generally be considered a primary concern of the referring agent.

The second stage, Dissonance, is marked by conflict and could be a gradual process. The conflict centers around one's beliefs that one's culture of origin, which is group deprecating (i.e., negative stereotypes/beliefs about one's own culture), is being challenged by opposing views that are positive. Eventually the individual will experience or encounter information that is inconsistent with his beliefs and attitudes about both his culture of origin and the dominant culture. To put it simply, a person experiences something inconsistent with his stereotypes about both groups that causes him to rethink his previously held beliefs. One of the most powerful ways that men are confronted with this is through a sudden encounter with racism. The example below helps to illustrate what happens during this stage.

A Hispanic male client once reported numerous stories in which he was not hired for jobs for which he was qualified. After numerous incidents of this hiring discrimination, he attempted to discuss the matter with an Anglo friend. Although his friend had accompanied him to a few of the job interviews, and even witnessed a hostile interaction with a prospective employer, his friend's responses were unsupportive, critical, and basically minimizing of the impact of these discriminatory incidents. Despondent and confused, the client decided to visit a vocational agency in a predominantly Hispanic neighborhood. Here the client had his experiences validated and was warmly received. This was reassuring and positive for him, yet left him conflicted since he had always idealized the Anglo community and devalued his community of origin.

The third stage, Resistance and Immersion, represents an almost complete turnaround from the Conformity Stage. The individual completely endorses minority-held views and rejects values of the dominant society and culture. What emerges is the strong desire to eliminate oppression directed toward minority groups, particularly his own. This desire seems fueled by three powerful feelings that an individual in this stage struggles to manage: Guilt, Shame, and Anger. Guilt and shame stem from beliefs that they in some way had been deceived or conned. Anger directed outward toward the dominant group provides a way of coping with these feelings; thus the newly acquired understanding of the social forces of oppression and racism become more evident. The question asked moves from "Who am I?" to "Why should I be ashamed of who I am?" The individual with originally low self-esteem is now actively challenged to raise it (Atkinson et al. 1989). Finally, it is also possible for overidealization to occur toward one's own group. A vignette illustrating this stage of identity development is presented below.

A Hispanic graduate student was referred to the counseling center of the university he attends. The presenting problem involved managing the stress of graduate school. The student reported constant heated arguments with professors and students about the pervasive racism present in his department and the curriculum. These arguments left him ostracized and labeled as "an angry Hispanic man." As a result, the student's academic performance suffered as well as his interpersonal relations. This student is clearly in the Resistance/Immersion stage in which he is endorsing minority-held views and rejecting the dominant culture. His newly awakened desire to eliminate oppression manifests as overt anger or passion for his newly adopted beliefs. The source of this passion may derive from guilt or shame for blindly accepting traditional teachings and not seeing the institutional racism that is now so clearly evident. The conflict for him is that he is still working within the dominant structure and trying to make changes in a system that is reluctant to change. His perceptions of racism are probably accurate and his anger is justified, yet when expressed, the system further alienates or blames him. New avenues for support are critical and additional strategies to manage the racist environment will need to be developed.

The fourth stage, Introspection, can be characterized as a time of confusion. Atkinson and colleagues (1989) believe that maintaining feelings of anger, guilt, and shame over time becomes psychologically draining and interferes with one's continued self-growth. A second component of this stage is the development of feelings of discontent or discomfort that may surface around the rigid views (e.g., all white people are bad) that an individual may currently hold toward both groups. Similar to what occurs in the earlier stages, individuals may encounter situations or people who do not fit their rigid views. For example, a Hispanic male may develop a friendship with a white person and discover that earlier beliefs about the individual's being a racist were inaccurate. This stage can easily be mistaken for Conformity; the critical difference lies in the absence of global racist self-hatred. Introspective clients do not hold internalized negative views toward themselves or other minority groups. The following example provides additional clarity.

A bisexual Hispanic HIV-impacted client began attending an HIV support group that was held in a minority-based community agency in a predominantly Hispanic neighborhood. At the meeting it was suggested by a fellow group member that he join him at another support group held in a predominantly Anglo gay health service organization. Initially reluctant about the prospect of going to a "white" HIV support group, he finally went; finding the experience to be positive, he connected with the members around similarities about HIV matters. This experience, while positive, left the man more confused. In this situation the client was comfortable in minority organizations but still held strong negative views toward white people. When confronted with a supportive group of white clients, it did not fit with his views and created confusion and a period of introspection for the client.

The final stage is Integrative Awareness, which is characterized by the ability to concurrently own and appreciate aspects of one's own culture as well as those of the United States culture at large. Past experiences of conflict and discomfort between the dominant culture and the minority group are now absent or greatly diminished. The individual is thus committed to eliminating all forms of oppression. During this evolutionary process, which occurs as one develops an inner sense of security and conflicts from previous stages become resolved, a belief emerges that there are acceptable and unacceptable aspects in all cultures and the culture should be examined before being accepted or rejected.

As outlined in Chapter 5, the above model is presented as a foundation upon which to build ideas about your clients' experience and manage issues surrounding ethnic and racial identity development. It is important to note that, as with most developmental models, there is always the possibility of great fluidity (i.e., an individual may vacillate from stage to stage) between and across stages, and individual variations cannot be ignored. Finally, it is important to note that an individual may have always been or may stay in one particular stage, such as Resistance/Immersion, and not necessarily experience subsequent stages.

Familialism

The importance of the family in relation to practical and emotional support is well documented in the psychological literature (Grebler et al. 1973, Heard 1982, Keitner et al. 1987). Familialism can be viewed as a cultural value that emphasizes the interdependency of the nuclear and extended family. This interdependence manifests itself around loyalty, reciprocity, feelings of obligation, and solidarity among family members. Mindel (1980) found that Hispanic families tend to have extensive interactions with relatives and may be more apt to turn to family rather than institutions for support. When a family member contracts HIV/AIDS, the cultural value of familialism is challenged. The question now becomes, How does HIV/AIDS impact Hispanic familialism?

This question can be examined from two perspectives: individual and family. At the individual or client level researchers have found that Hispanic men were less likely than whites to disclose their serostatus to families and friends (Mason et al. 1995), primarily out of concern for protecting parents. This study also demonstrated that Hispanics were also less likely than whites to disclose gay or bisexual orientation and that disclosure was moderated by level of acculturation. Less acculturated Hispanics revealed fewer aspects of their sexual orientation than their counterparts who were more highly acculturated. Delayed disclosure results in limited opportunity for familial support. The decision not to disclose appears to be a painful internal struggle the client usually faces alone. The desire not to disclose to parents or siblings stems from the wish to protect the family from additional hardships or to avoid having the family worry about something they cannot control or possibly understand. Moreover, for Hispanic men who have sex with men, disclosing one's HIV status may result in the reluctant disclosure of other aspects of their identity that have previously been compartmentalized or fragmented. This may be particularly true for the married bisexual Hispanic male or the Hispanic male with a concealed history of injection drug use. Clearly, motives for nondisclosure vary. Exploration of each client's motives for nondisclosure should be identified, and irrational beliefs or fears should be emphatically confronted. For example, a Hispanic male may not tell his family for fear of being asked to leave the home. While this possibility exists, its likelihood is uncertain and seems, from my clinical experience, to be minimal due to the fact that the client is still "part of the family." I have also observed that clients who report not disclosing to protect the family upon closer exploration may be protecting themselves against having to confront powerful feelings (e.g., fear or shame) associated with integrating HIV into their lives. Finally, it is important to note that intrapsychic reasons such as high levels of denial ("If I don't tell anyone, then I don't have AIDS") may also be operating, but it is usually the psychological reasons that are emphasized at the expense of exploring the cultural aspects associated with nondisclosure.

At the family level the question that must be asked is How is the family supportive? Given the stigma associated with HIV/AIDS and the limited or inaccurate knowledge of AIDS that

Hispanics may have, when it enters the family unconditional support may not be guaranteed. Instead, concern for other family members may take precedence over the client's needs. Again, the desire to protect the family may be predominant and play itself out around fear of contagion, particularly with children. This may be done covertly or out of fear rather than malice. For example, a Hispanic client of mine once reported that his sister, after becoming aware of his HIV status, became visibly uncomfortable when he tried to play with his nephew. Of course, this would never be acknowledged or discussed. The need to maintain smooth relations (Simpatia) may lead to culturally sanctioned secrets within the family that may leave everyone struggling in silence and not accessing emotional support from each other. Family therapy is a useful treatment modality for the Hispanic family confronting AIDS. It is important to assess the family dynamics, especially if your client still lives at home or plans to return home due to failing health or economic hardship. In situations of return, anticipatory planning or educational family sessions can be an invaluable asset. On a positive note, when Hispanic families are successfully able to manage the challenge of HIV to the family, the strength and nurturance that the client can receive from the family is overwhelming and powerful.

Religion

Religion is a core institutional structure held in virtually all Hispanic cultures. Broadly speaking, Roman Catholicism is the predominant institution that pervades the individual and collective psyches of Latino cultures. This religion, which is based upon a conservative and fundamentally evangelical tradition of Judeo-Christian values, strongly rejects homosexuality as a legitimate lifestyle and holds critical views toward illicit drug use.

For most Hispanics the church, whether it be Roman Catholic, Methodist, or other mainstream faiths, is a major source of emotional support around times of conflict or crisis. For the gay/bisexual or drug-using Hispanic, access to this support system may be impeded. The church (minister, priest, or general community of family) may be rejecting or hostile. The dilemma or psychological conflict that may arise for the gay/bisexual Hispanic can be emotionally overwhelming. If the family system is contextually very religious, this religiosity unconsciously fosters a wall of alienation separating the client from his family. Secrecy and selective disclosure hinder any possibility of deep, intimate, and meaningful support. For example, a gay Hispanic client of mine reported growing frustration with his family, who indicated that they were "praying for him." At first those words were comforting, but as time passed it became less clear whether his family was praying because he had sinned and was in desperate need of forgiveness or whether they were praying for him to regain his health. This ambiguity caused a great deal of sadness and isolation for the client; thus he and many Hispanic men are often left spiritually isolated with limited access to important sources of solace: family and church.

Careful assessment of how the gay or bisexual male is experiencing his spirituality is important. Some clients report that when returning to the Roman Catholic church they've been told that they are evil sinners and should beg forgiveness. To compensate for these traditional shortcomings, it is important to originate a referral to a culturally and theologically competent pastoral care worker familiar with the population and the dilemma of HIV infection. In situations where respectful and unconditional support and empathy is offered by clergy, clients seem to flourish. When this type of support is not available, it may be important for the therapist to work with clients to help redefine or reclaim their spirituality. Toward the latter stages of AIDS, when spiritual issues are often raised and internal conflicts seem evident, the source of these conflicts should be identified and resolution should be attempted. I have seen much guilt, shame, and remorse reported by Hispanic male clients. These affects emerge from feelings that they somehow weren't "good enough." Specifically, not a good enough husband, provider, student, son, and so on. This low self-worth may be tied to goals they set for themselves that they never accomplished due to obstacles beyond their control. The shame or remorse is often associated with how they manage their guilt (substance use, anonymous sexual encounters, violence) about not being good enough. These emotions often make the client feel as though he may be unworthy of "going to heaven" or may need to be punished for his mistakes. Treatment that focuses on providing a cognitive understanding as well as an empathic ear will allow thorough exploration of these issues, with the goal a resolution that may not be self-punitive.

Individual Considerations

Hispanics in this country are not a homogeneous group. Between- and within-group differences exist. Consideration of individual variations is critical for successful treatment of the Hispanic male. Specific areas in which individual variation occurs are discussed below.

Sexual Identity Development

Given that over 52 percent of the Hispanics contracting AIDS report having same-gender sexual relations, it is important for practitioners to have a clear understanding of the variation in sexual identity development for Hispanic men and its implications for psychological distress. Troiden (1993) views sexual identity as something that is incorporated into one's self-concept similar to other aspects of one's identity (e.g., gender or ethnicity). It is this incorporation or how one manages to integrate or *not* integrate this aspect (same-gender relations) that needs to be understood by both the client and the clinician. The research cited earlier by Carballo-Dieguez and Dolezal (1994a) lends support to the belief that various levels of integration of same-sex behaviors exist. Hispanic men who have sex with men often do not identify as gay or bisexual and often report that their sexual relations with men are just acts that do not make them homosexual. They may attribute situational factors for their behaviors as opposed to integrating that behavior into their sense of self. Even when there is an acknowledgment that one is bisexual or gay, resolution of the sexual conflicts or psychological distress cannot be immediately assumed. For most gay and bisexual men, management of sexual identity is a lifelong process that is mediated by the degree of internalized homophobia an individual may have adopted. *Internalized homophobia* can be defined as the negative feelings an individual holds about being gay or bisexual, which often are a reflection of the degree to which they have accepted the pejorative attitudes and attributions society in general holds toward homosexuality.

Within Hispanic communities the negative outlook toward homosexuality is more severe than in the general society. This may be due to the culture's strong religious influences and the rigid gender sex roles that the culture adopts. To be homosexual is strongly identified with being female or effeminate; in fact, in some respects homosexuality is even mildly tolerated if it stays within an effeminate context. This is evidenced by the presence of female impersonators in some of the more popular Spanish-language television shows. Nonetheless, clinicians need to be mindful of the negative psychological consequences associated with unresolved sexual identity conflicts experienced by Hispanic men. The most negative psychological conflict appears to be a fragmented sense of self, in which the emotions associated with same-gender sexual relationships are intolerable and cut off from how they see themselves as individuals. The few emotions experienced are usually negative or shameful and are quickly repressed. Treatment should focus on identifying for the client how he manages homophobia and determining whether his coping strategies are psychologically healthy. If they are not, more adaptive ways of coping need to be developed. The therapist can help the client explore possible new strategies. It has been my experience that utilizing community resources such as gay Hispanic organizations (which have formed or are forming in most urban settings) can be very useful. These organizations provide opportunities for clients to see the various ways other Hispanic gay and bisexual men have successfully managed the internal and external assaults to their self-esteem. Referrals of this nature are valuable adjuncts to treatment.

Childhood Sexual Abuse

Male sex abuse is an area that has been given little attention in the psychological literature (Lew 1990). As this hidden epidemic begins to reveal itself, its psychological ramifications become evident. Recent research by Carballo-Dieguez and Dolezal (1994b) suggests that past history of childhood sexual abuse can serve as a marker to identify men at greater risk for HIV. In their study using a cohort of 182 Puerto Rican men who have sex with men, they differentiated three groups: (1) an abused group (had sex before age 13 with males four years their senior) in which men felt hurt by the experience or were unwilling participants; (2) a willing/not hurt abused group, who reported not being hurt by the experience; and (3) a no-older-partner group in which no abuse occurred, or if they had sex before age 13 it was with someone less than four years their senior. These results revealed that the men in the abused group were significantly more likely than men in the no-older-partner group to engage in unsafe receptive anal sex, with age and level of education serving as moderating cofactors. Specifically, less educated and older men had more unprotected receptive anal intercourse. This study is important for a variety of reasons. First, it raises the issue of sexual abuse in men, which is a neglected area of study. Second, it was conducted using an exclusively Hispanic sample. Third, it shows a relationship between childhood sexual abuse and HIV. Fourth, the study has significant prevention implications. The utility of this study for clinicians focuses around raising awareness of the need to conduct a thorough assessment of past history of sexual abuse. Special attention must be given to the patient's management of the psychological traumas associated with past sexual abuse, especially since the abuse may put them at greater risk for self-destructive behavior. Although a discussion of the treatment of survivors of male sexual abuse is beyond the scope of this chapter, identifying the issue is critical in developing an appropriate treatment plan. Finally, while the aforementioned study was conducted on a sample of men who have sex with men, it would be naive to assume that Hispanic heterosexual men may not have been impacted negatively by a past trauma of abuse, given that other research (Hunter 1990) indicates that male sexual abuse often goes underreported.

Immigration Status

Differences in immigrant status among clients are crucial issues that one needs to be aware of when working with Hispanics. Hispanics who are undocumented United States residents have additional stressors to contend with besides issues of HIV disease. They are likely to be more guarded and less disclosing of personal information. In these situations, development of a trusting working relationship must be paramount for successful interventions to be achieved. A key to that trust is communicating to the client the confidential nature of the therapeutic relationship. Given the recent political climate and changes in society's views toward undocu-mented residents (as evidenced by the passage of Proposition 187 in California), establishing trust will be an even greater challenge. The additional economic hurdle that many gay and bisexual Hispanics face from being undocumented can lead to male prostitution as an economic option. Finally, the taking of a wealthy Anglo lover can be another option utilized to contend with economic hardship. This has been observed in undocumented as well as legal residents. This is sometimes referred to as the "benefactor" syndrome.

Maladaptive Coping

As with any irritant, individuals cope with stress in adaptive or maladaptive ways. Common maladaptive strategies observed in working with Hispanic men have included substance use, denial, compartmentalization, and suicide. Special attention should be given to the manner in which HIV-impacted Hispanic men are coping with the virus; maladaptive approaches should be sensitively, directly challenged and more adaptive approaches should be offered to replace them.

In some respects, alcohol and drug use are often a socially sanctioned way of coping with strong affect. It is not uncommon for Hispanic men to get together for a weekend evening with the purpose of getting drunk. Also, drugs and alcohol excuse or provide a way of dissociating the undesirable behaviors (e.g., same-sex relations or unsafe sex practices) from being part of who they are. Instead, they may blame the behaviors on drugs or alcohol. Clinicians should carefully assess frequency and patterns of alcohol or substance use and clients should be counseled as to the increased risk the client may be placing himself in regard to reexposure to HIV.

Denial is a very common defense mechanism that has adaptive aspects (healthy denial) and negative aspects. The clinician should carefully assess where along the denial continuum the Hispanic male client falls. The burden of machismo for the Hispanic male may lead some to deny that they are experiencing any emotional distress, rather that they are handling the crisis "like a man." A clinician can confront the denial by reframing what it means to be a man, that is, part of being a man is being responsible for one's own health and the health of others, which means seeking out assistance and support when needed. I have found that broadening the definition of masculinity to incorporate self-care components has met with significant success with Hispanic male clients living with HIV disease.

Compartmentalization can loosely be defined as coping with conflicts by taking aspects of your life and sharply separating them out or not integrating them into who you are. An example is developing different sets of friends and making sure they don't meet, or doing your "family things" on Sundays, your "work things" on Fridays, and your "gay things" on Saturdays. It is important to realize that this type of behavior is done by all of us in some fashion. The issue here is the degree or severity of compartmentalization. Integrating HIV into one's life is particularly difficult given the nature of the disease progression and the stigma associated with it.

Using compartmentalization as a way of coping with HIV is especially likely if this type of coping has been used before with other aspects of one's identity. For example, a Hispanic man who has sex with men may often compartmentalize this "secret" part of his life and may try the same strategy with HIV. The strategy is only partially successful and leaves the client isolated and with limited support. Shame and guilt appear to be the major affective states that clients attempt to avoid in these situations.

Finally, suicide risk is always an issue for anyone infected with HIV. Research suggests that men successfully commit suicide at higher rates than do women; thus suicide should be assessed throughout treatment.

Progression of HIV

Clinicians may begin treatment of the HIV client anywhere along the spectrum of HIV disease. It is important to have a clear understanding of where an individual may be along the line of progression. At each stage the clinician should ask him- or herself the following question: To what degree are overarching cultural constructs impacting the client's management of HIV at this point in the illness? At various points along the HIV spectrum certain cultural constructs take on greater significance. For example, at the later stages of HIV, religion and/or spirituality often become a salient consideration for the client. Likewise, familial concerns may become greater when the client is no longer able to work. In the earlier stages of the illness issues of acculturation or sexual identity may be more paramount. Each individual is different and thus each cultural construct should be carefully examined. The clinical case vignette presented below will assist the reader in integrating the issues covered in this chapter.

José is a 24-year-old Hispanic gay male who has been living with his partner for several years. He is of slight build, neatly groomed and soft-spoken. He was born and raised in Ecuador, and he identified himself as Catholic. He reports being diagnosed HIV-positive while still living in his country of origin. After the diagnosis he worked on a cruise ship for about a year while trying to find a way to enter the United States. José entered the country as an undocumented resident in 1988. It appears that he fled his country as a way of trying to run away from his HIV status and to live an openly gay lifestyle. He reports coming out in Ecuador. There he would meet men in the streets and engage in numerous sexual encounters. He exhibited remorse and shame when discussing his early sexual history. José was raised primarily by his mother and reports his father may have had a history of mental illness.

When José arrived in the United States, he lived in Tampa for a while, then eventually moved to the Midwest where he stayed with an uncle for nine months, after which he moved in with an Anglo lover. While living in the United States he worked as a busboy at several restaurants. José did not seek any medical treatment until August of 1993. At that time he began exhibiting symptoms of HIV infection. At his first medical visit he learned his CD-4 count was 44 (the norm is 800–1,200). Not surprisingly, he began showing signs of depression, specifically, decreased appetite, weight loss, sleep disturbance, and a general feeling of anhedonia. He reported increased desire to seek out anonymous sexual encounters. He would find himself going to adult bookstores and engaging in such encounters. Afterwards he would feel a great deal of shame and remorse but couldn't stop going. José also reports using marijuana on a regular basis.

Since beginning medical treatment, José's condition has declined. He has had numerous hospitalizations that have exacerbated his depressive symptoms, and he was diagnosed with Cytomegalovirus retinitis, which often results in blindness.

The aforementioned case illustrates the complexity of issues that are usually present with this population. To minimize confusion, it is best to take each issue individually. First, in regard to his male identity development, José did not display rigid male socialization. Instead, he appeared boyish in both his physical presentation and his manner of relating to others. This may be related to his youth. Second, in regard to ethnic identity, José appeared to be in the Conformity Stage. This is evidenced by his idealization of the United States as the land of opportunity. When he arrived he sought relationships predominantly with Anglo men and moved into a gay ghetto as soon as he was financially able. He also spoke negatively of his country of origin and gave no indication of wanting to return should his health deteriorate.

Third, psychological management of his HIV status appeared to have been difficult for José. He coped with the initial diagnosis of HIV by "fleeing" or going into denial about the need for medical monitoring. As a result, his condition progressed at a rapid pace. His initial means of coping with the virus indicated that he was overwhelmed by stressful information and had not developed adaptive ways of dealing with stress. Since beginning treatment, José experienced several events that moved him along the progression of HIV at a rapid pace. Specifically, his CD-4 count declined enough to warrant an AIDS diagnosis, and he had multiple hospitalizations and is now struggling with long-term chronic illness (CMV).

Clearly this was not a linear progression. These events were rapid in onset and concurrent, and the stress resulted in increased depressive symptomatology. Establishing support was challenging as most of his family lived out of the country and the patient was undocumented. Medical evaluation was strongly indicated and suicidal ideation was evaluated.

Finally, José's increased desire for anonymous sexual encounters appeared to be another form of escape as well as an area in which he had in the past felt good about himself. He reported that his "looks are all he has" and he felt good when others found him desirable. This also suggested a degree of machismo in relation to his need for sexual accomplishments, which raised his self-worth. The fear that he was slowly losing his machismo was very frightening to him. The conflict he experienced involved the guilt and shame he felt when he deceived his lover. Also, his high level of religiosity contributed to this shame around HIV and his sexuality, about which his family was unaware. All these issues were discussed in treatment and alternative ways of coping were established.

REFERENCES

Atkinson, D. R., Morten, G., and Sue, D. (1989). *Counseling American Minorities: A Cross Cultural Perspective.* Dubuque, IA: Wm. C. Brown.

Bernal, G., and Knight, M., eds. (1993). *Ethnic Identity: Formation and Tranmission among Hispanics and Other Minorities.* Albany: State University of New York Press.

Bing, E., and Soto, T. (1991). Treatment issues for African-Americans and Hispanics with AIDS. *Psychiatric Medicine* Vol. 9, 3:455–467.

Carballo-Dieguez, A. (1989). Hispanic culture, gay male culture and AIDS: counseling implications. *Journal of Counseling and Development*, Vol. 68:26–30.

Carballo-Dieguez, A., and Dolezal, C. (1994a). Contrasting types of Puerto Rican men who have sex with men. *Journal of Psychology & Human Sexuality* 6(4):41–67.

———— (1994b). Association between history of childhood sexual abuse and adult HIV-risk sexual behavior in Puerto Rican men who have sex with men. *Child Abuse and Neglect*, Vol. 19, 5, 595–605.

Carrier, J. M. (1985). Mexican male bisexuality. *Journal of Homosexuality* 11(1):75–85.

Centers for Disease Control and Prevention (CDC). (1995). *HIV/AIDS Surveillance Report* 7, No. 1, 11–21.

Eisler, R. M., and Skidmore, J. R. (1987). Masculine gender role stress: scale development and component factors in the appraisal of stressful situations. *Behavior Modification* 11:123–136.

Flannery, J. G. (1978). Alexithymia, II. The association with unexplained physical distress. *Psychotherapy and Psychosomatics* 30:193–197.

Grebler, L., Moore, J. W., and Guzman, R. K. (1973). The family: variation in time and space. In *Introduction to Chicano Studies*, ed. L. I. Duran and H. R. Bernard, pp. 309–331. New York: Macmillan.

Heard, D. (1982). Family systems and the attachment dynamic. *Journal of Family Therapy* 4:99–116.

Hunter, M. (1990). *Abused Boys: The Neglected Victims of Sexual Abuse.* New York: Fawcett Columbine.

Keitner, G., Miller, I. W., Epstein, A. E., et al. (1987). Family functioning and the course of major depression. *Comprehensive Psychiatry* 28:54–64.

Levinson, D. (1978). *Seasons of a Man's Life.* New York: Knopf.

Lew, M. (1990). *Victims No Longer: Men Recovering from Incest and Other Sexual Abuse.* New York: HarperCollins.

Marin, G. (1989). AIDS prevention among Hispanics: needs, risk behaviors and cultural values. *Public Health Reports* 104:411–415.

Mason, H., Marks, G., Simoni, J. R., et al. (1995). Culturally sanctioned secrets? Latino men's nondisclosure of HIV infection to family, friends, and lovers. *Health Psychology* 14:1, 6–12.

Mindel, C. H. (1980). Extended familialism among urban Mexican-American, Anglos and blacks. *Hispanic Journal of Behavioral Science* 2:21–34.

Pennebaker, J. W. (1992). Inhibition as the linchpin of health. In *Hostility, Coping, and Health*, ed. H. S. Friedman. Washington, DC: American Psychological Association.

Sutkin, L. F., and Good, G. (1987). Therapy with men in health-care settings. In *Handbook of Counseling and Psychotherapy with Men*, ed. M. Scher, M. Stevens, G. Good, and G. A. Eichenfield, pp. 372–387. Newbury Park, CA: Sage.

Troiden, R. R. (1993). The formation of homosexual identities. In *Psychological Perspectives on Lesbian and Gay Male Experiences*, ed. L. D. Garnets and D. C. Kimmel, pp. 191–217. New York: Columbia University Press.

7

HIV Disease and Women

DOREEN SALINA, ANDREA HAMILTON, AND
CATHERINE LEAKE

Women are increasingly at risk for AIDS, and mental health professionals will be increasingly involved in the care of these women. When AIDS was initially identified, it was conceptualized by both the medical community and society as a disorder that impacted gay men primarily. Medical and psychological understanding of the syndrome was limited, and its impact on women and girls was not studied, partially because of the low numbers of women diagnosed with AIDS in the early stages of the epidemic. Lack of knowledge regarding women and AIDS has reflected in part the epidemiological course of the disease in the United States as well as the traditional trend in Western medicine to study disease with male patients and generalize those findings to women. Because AIDS was first identified and diagnosed in homosexual males, the cause and impact of the disease quickly became associated with the gay male lifestyle. This excluded women from being seen as a population at risk and fostered in them a false sense of safety.

At the outset of the epidemic, public health messages focused on educating individuals about how HIV was transmitted. This consisted primarily of identifying routes of transmission and encouraging condom usage to reduce the risk of HIV, the agent believed to cause AIDS. These early messages were designed to identify and manage early signs of the disease through changing male behaviors. Public health officials did not tailor these messages for the specific constraints society and culture place on women that increase their risk of contracting HIV.

As a result of this neglect, over the last decade there has been a dramatic increase in AIDS cases among women and children since its identification as a disease entity. The numbers of women diagnosed with AIDS is growing at an alarming rate. As of June 1995, 64,822 girls and women have been diagnosed with AIDS (CDC 1995). This does not include the number of girls under the age of 13 who are diagnosed HIV positive through birth to an infected mother or through breast feeding. Through June 1995, 6,611 children have been diagnosed with AIDS, and this trend increases with each reporting of the cumulative AIDS statistics (CDC 1995). Approximately 81 percent of women with AIDS are between the ages of 20 and 44 at diagnosis; 62 percent of these women are between the ages of 20 and 39, the primary child-bearing years. African-American women comprise 52 percent of women with AIDS; 19 percent are Latina.

In addition to women formally diagnosed with AIDS in this country, there are significant numbers (16,642) identified as HIV positive who do not meet full criteria for an AIDS diagnosis. Sexual transmission between heterosexuals is the most prevalent mode of HIV transmission among women (34 percent). Twenty-seven percent of HIV-infected women report contracting the virus through intravenous (IV) drug use (CDC 1995). This trend is consistent across all racial/ethnic groups. Given that the majority of the women in this country are unaware of their HIV status, the magnitude of HIV infection is likely to be much greater than has been documented.

Sensitivity to the psychological, cultural, and familial impact

HIV has upon women has been woefully neglected in the psychological treatment literature. Many of the issues and challenges confronted by HIV-impacted women are discussed below. In addition, treatment strategies and approaches are offered to mental health professionals working with this population. These include (1) helping women access and utilize effective and life-prolonging care; (2) addressing the concerns of family members, especially children; (3) preventing transmission to sexual partners; and providing support for women experiencing the psychological consequences of having an illness for which there is no cure.

HIV ANTIBODY TESTING AND WOMEN

Even when women suspect that they are HIV-infected because of their high-risk behaviors, many—especially those who are asymptomatic—are extremely reluctant to obtain HIV antibody testing. There are many reasons for this. Often women are afraid to have their suspicions confirmed; others believe that if they are HIV-infected, confirmation of their positive status will do no good as there is no cure for AIDS.

Many women lack access to accurate information and quality health care, which contributes to their being misinformed about HIV antibody testing and increases their anxiety about undergoing the testing procedure. Some women are reluctant to be tested because it may confirm that their sexual partner has been engaging in unsafe behaviors, including sexual relations with other individuals. Others fear that as a consequence of being identified as HIV positive their families will be stigmatized. Mental health professionals must be cognizant of these issues and spend time assisting women in their decision-making process. Counseling should take place before antibody testing and a coping plan designed to foster the most adaptive response to the test results must be developed.

Without trained counselors to explain the benefits of receiving HIV antibody testing, some women may be unable to understand how an early diagnosis can help increase the quality and quantity of their lives should they be HIV positive. Why testing is important should be fully explained and any fears the woman has should be addressed directly. Removing the mystery should be considered one of the primary counseling tasks of the mental health professional at this juncture.

The reader is encouraged to conduct a thorough diagnostic assessment of suicidal or homicidal potential and the need to monitor the client's mood during the therapeutic relationship. If the client is treated immediately after confirmation of an HIV-positive diagnosis, she may be immobilized by guilt and fear. At this point, the mental health professional has an excellent opportunity to link the woman with various community resources and monitor her compliance with recommended treatment. The mental health professional should work on developing trust with the woman to help facilitate medical compliance such as taking medication, eating properly, and enrolling in a drug/alcohol rehabilitation program if it is indicated. The emotional sequelae of an HIV-positive diagnosis can be devastating. The types of feelings that accompany this diagnosis vary, but generally entail disbelief, denial, anger, and sadness. Therapists should attempt to create a safe and open atmosphere that will allow the client to express her feelings and feel supported.

ISSUES FACED BY WOMEN WITH AIDS

Women with HIV/AIDS face many of the same issues that others with AIDS confront. Besides fearing death and dying, multiple bereavement is common and may include losses of health, future aspirations, and sexual expression. Their sense of invulnerability and physical desirability may disappear along with financial security. Losses of friends, lovers, and spouses who have already died may cause additional grief. Fears that a partner may abandon them or guilt over exposing a partner to the virus often emerge. The disease raises existential issues about the quality and meaning of life, loneliness, and isolation (Winiarski 1991). Suicidal ideation is also frequently observed (Dworkin and Pincu 1993).

Women have some unique psychological challenges as well. These difficulties may include grief over the loss of childbearing potential and the burden of making decisions about maintaining a pregnancy or the care of dependent children. These resolutions must often be made quickly as evidence indicates that women die more quickly than men after a diagnosis of AIDS (Ybarra 1991). This finding may be attributable to several factors. Women appear to be more likely than men to get opportunistic infections such as Pneumocystis carinii pneumonia (PCP), whereas men appear more likely to get Kaposi's sarcoma, a cancer that offers a longer prognosis than other AIDS-related illnesses (Shaw 1987). Women are also discriminated against in the health care system. As late as 1992 women composed only 6–7 percent of 7,659 patients in antiviral drug clinical trials (Pizzi 1992). Moreover, women were initially excluded from participating in tests of zidovudine (AZT) and didioxyinosine (DDI), drugs commonly prescribed for HIV-impacted people. Instead they received these drugs absent research to determine effective dosages and possible side effects specific to women (Pizzi 1992).

Another explanation for the shorter survival times is that many women are diagnosed later. Many discover their seropositive status when they learn they are pregnant; others at the birth of an infected child (Pizzi 1992); still others after another crisis, such as rape (Sherr et al. 1993). In these cases women may not be prepared psychologically for their diagnosis. Women caring for an infected child must plan the child's medical care and access to school (Ybarra 1991). Many women at this time are grappling simultaneously with feelings of guilt as they watch their child die; many fear loss of custody of their children should their seropositive status be revealed. While all of this is under way, women are confronted with having to negotiate alternative lifestyle changes (e.g., financial, social, and sexual).

PSYCHOLOGICAL TREATMENT OF WOMEN WITH HIV DISEASE

Mental health professionals have multiple tasks when working with women with HIV infection. The therapist may be the first person the woman informs about her HIV status and engagement in high-risk behaviors. How the therapist responds is extremely important as this response is the woman's first indicator of what type of reaction she may expect from others. The mental health professional must examine her or his personal belief systems thoroughly and be aware of countertransference issues that may be stimulated by issues raised by the client; the many prejudicial attitudes infected individuals often face from family, friends, and medical personnel mandate that she feel supported and accepted in experiencing her feelings and making decisions that are right for her. This can be facilitated by the therapist's directly discussing the woman's fears regarding her HIV status, using language most familiar to her. While some therapists' psychological paradigms may discourage the direct bringing up of pertinent issues, for a woman with HIV disease this approach can be inappropriate. The mental health professional must assume an active role in helping the woman sort out her concerns and formulate action plans to meet her goals. He or she must foster an open and supportive environment that will allow the client to process her emotions, clarify her thoughts, and make informed, rational decisions.

During this first phase, there may be a need for frequent sessions and immediate connection with social service agencies that provide assistance, particularly social support or self-help groups. A team approach to assist the woman in accepting her diagnosis is recommended when possible. While the therapist can focus on the affective conflicts and help their clients plan for the future, support groups consisting of other women living with HIV/AIDS may help to reduce feelings of hopelessness and isolation and present a more positive and realistic perspective on how to live with AIDS. They can also provide valuable practical information and assistance for the woman with children as she confronts the challenges that HIV presents to her and her family.

The next phase generally centers on decisions the woman is forced to make. Many women are initially immobilized and unable to take self-protective action. The therapist should attempt to create a supportive environment that will facilitate the woman's acceptance of her HIV status by allowing her to grieve and express her feelings. The next therapeutic task should be to help her identify what she feels she needs or wants to do to create the most positive experiences she can for herself and significant others. This process will differ across women depending on individual circumstances and health status. The issues that often come up at this time include developing and maintaining a medical treatment regime, identifying which members of her social support network she wants to inform of her HIV-positive status, and how she wants to go about that process. Reproductive issues and future care of children will also need to be addressed.

LIVING WITH HIV/AIDS

Sex and the HIV-Infected Woman

Many women, once identified as HIV positive, erroneously believe they can no longer engage in sexual activity. This fear may keep them from receiving treatment or disclosing their positive status to their sexual partners. Mental health professionals should be knowledgeable about sexual behaviors that entail little or no risk of HIV transmission. ACT UP, a national advocacy group developed to address the AIDS crisis through community activism, defines safer sex as "a way of taking control of, and taking responsibility for, one's sexual behavior" (ACT UP/NY 1990). Safer sex behaviors prescribed include any act of sexual intimacy in which blood, semen, or vaginal secretions are not exchanged between partners. This may include "dry sex" options such as masturbation, exhibitionism, voyeurism, fantasy, talking, massage, or frotteurism. It also includes "wet sex" options in which barriers such as latex condoms with Nonoxynol-9 lubricant, dental dams, heavy-gauge plastic wrap, latex surgical gloves, or finger cots prevent the possible exchanges of blood, semen, or vaginal secretions. ACT UP recommends these products be used with any sexual act that includes the possibility of an exchange of bodily fluids, including oral, anal, and vaginal sex; sadomasochism; bondage; and finger penetration of the vagina or anus.

Mental health professionals working with clients impacted by HIV must be knowledgeable and comfortable discussing the aforementioned sexual activities and safer sex practices with their clients. Fostering an open and nonjudgmental atmosphere is crucial. Therapists should use language the client is familiar with and understands. Technical terms should be explained and the therapist who does not fully comprehend terms the client uses should seek clarification from the client.

Several studies (Brown 1990, Quadagno et al. 1991) indicate that although informed about safer sex techniques, many women do not implement them consistently. What are the barriers to women's effective use of safer sex techniques? One may be that women are often more concerned with the level of intimacy achieved during sex than the actual penetration. This frequently places the woman in conflict with male partners who may resist behaviors that do not involve penetration and that may violate cultural norms regarding sexual behavior. While safer sex behaviors help prevent HIV transmission, they may not be deemed acceptable in some cultures for some women and men (Mays and Cochran 1988). Religious, peer, or subcultural constraints regarding birth control methods often conflict with safer sex behaviors (e.g., use of condoms) for Latinos and other racial/ethnic minorities (Mays and Cochran 1988, Wermuth et al. 1991).

In addition to individual and cultural constraints, many women experience low self-efficacy in relation to male partners and feel ill prepared to maintain control over their sexual behavior, especially in cultures in which the man's desires take priority (Ickovics et al. 1994). This presents a particularly difficult atmosphere in which to engage in self-protective behaviors. Insisting on a male partner's use of condoms requires partner cooperation and communication techniques that successfully influence this behavior. To initiate consistent condom use and other safer-sex practices, however, women must introduce acts that may be viewed as promoting separateness and distrust. The mental health professional must address these attitudes, preferably with both partners, to ensure that they understand that engaging in safer-sex techniques does not mean "no sex" or "boring sex" or suggest a lack of love or commitment between partners. Many couples will resist such techniques in the (erroneous) belief that as they are both infected, there is no need. Several studies have shown that repeated exposure to HIV causes additional, unwanted symptoms and may hasten the progression of HIV disease (Van De Wijgert et al. 1993). Consequently, therapists should periodically ask their HIV-positive clients about their use of safer-sex techniques and encourage them to continue to protect their health. If a therapist discovers that a client is routinely not practicing safer sex, examining the feelings, thoughts, and factors associated with the unsafe sexual activity is strongly indicated.

THE INTERACTION OF FEMALE GENDER ROLE SOCIALIZATION AND HIV

While early AIDS-prevention messages and interventions focused primarily on high-risk behaviors associated with HIV transmission with respect to gay men, women were largely ignored as a target audience and the roles of gender and culture were not addressed. This situation resulted from a lack of understanding of how individual belief systems, sex role expectations, and specific cultural values impact upon women's behaviors associated with transmission. While women continued to lead lives believing they were not at risk, they were, in fact, especially vulnerable to the virus. Their vulnerability in many ways is promoted by social conditions that define and limit the power of women in mainstream culture (Chodorow 1989). In some minority cultures these conditions can render the woman powerless to protect herself or inhibit her ability to seek treatment due to cultural sanctions (Ickovics et al. 1994). Social factors, such as the way in which women are taught to behave, diminish many women's ability to protect themselves. Examples of these social factors include (1) the socialization of women to maintain relationships at the expense of their own needs; (2) stigmatizing and punishing women who are assertive in their communications and behavior patterns; and (3) indoctrinating women to believe they are unable to influence behavior change in others, particularly men.

Many women feel discomfort in discussing sex with their therapists or their sexual partners. Many have been socialized to experience embarrassment and inhibition with respect to their own sexual desires (Tolman 1991). As a result, there is a double standard in mainstream society between males and females when it comes to initiating sexual contact. Many women may feel that initiating discussions about sex with a prospective partner is tantamount to inviting sexual activity at that moment, and subsequently feel discomfort at assuming a dominant sexual role. Many women may be influenced by societal norms that equate overt sexuality with a "bad girl" image: "good girls" do not initiate talk about sex or instigate sexual activity. Unlike their male counterparts, women have not been socialized to carry condoms for unexpected sexual encounters. Collectively, these challenges can be overwhelming to many women and it is understandable why some may be very informed about HIV and safer-sex techniques, but unable to use their knowledge and implement these techniques.

Generally, women are socialized to play more passive roles than men (Chodorow 1989). Relationships are of primary importance, and women remain the primary caregivers, often placing the needs of others above their own. In some cases this means relinquishing self-protective barriers in favor of maintaining relational ties at all costs. Without diminishing the importance of women's values, the fact remains that their roles and the social conditions that maintain them facilitate HIV infection and often prevent women from receiving early treatment.

Cognitive behavioral techniques have been successful in empowering women, teaching them through assertiveness training and role playing to state their needs and protect themselves and their partners (e.g., "I love you, but if we can't use a condom, we can't have intercourse" [Jemott et al. 1992]). Homework assignments (e.g., labeling and expressing feelings and thoughts, limit setting, meditation and relaxation training) that require the use of these newly developed skills will enhance the woman's ability to use them at critical junctures. The client who experiences successful outcomes with the homework assignments will have a clearer perception of her own self-efficacy and be better prepared to implement these skills in the more difficult sexual arena.

Therapists may next want to consider practicing "no condom, no sex communication" exercises with the client. This approach involves having the therapist model the client's role (i.e., communicate to her partner the "no condom, no sex" ground rules) while the client role-plays her partner. The client can act out her worst-case scenario—insisting on the use of a condom. Through the therapist's modeling of the woman's role, the client can gain competency as well as clarify the motivation of her worst fears regarding insistence on safer-sex behaviors.

When both partners are infected, the woman will usually address the needs of her partner and/or children before she cares for her own health needs. This can be manifested in many ways, such as choosing to comply with the male partner's expectations rather than securing rest or care. Many women feel they have no power when confronted with the male's expectation that she continue to fulfill her role despite her deteriorating health status. The mental health professional can be useful in seeing both parties in couple's therapy and discussing the pertinent issues. A plan can be developed to address possible role conflicts, power differentials, and distribution of household chores and tasks across all family members, and to schedule important "downtime" for the HIV-impacted family member. Linkage with other HIV/AIDS social service agencies may also provide the woman and her family with additional resources that may ease the burdens of her and her family. This linkage is especially critical to low-income women who have access to few resources, including adequate health care and medication. Consequently, mental health professionals working with HIV-impaired women will need to become comfortable about occasionally serving as case manager for their clients. Flexibility on the part of the therapist is an essential element to the effective treatment of clients living with HIV.

Ethnic/Lifestyle/Age Differences in HIV-Infected Women

Mays and Cochran (1988) state that we must not underestimate the variety of ethnic, racial, socioeconomic, cultural, and religious factors that influence sexual behavior patterns. They suggest that for poor women sex may function as a source of employment or as a way to acquire emotional support. For some women the risk of being alone or unsuccessful in relationships may seem greater than the risk of contracting HIV. Furthermore, Mays and Cochran (1988) report that a small subset of women experience verbal and physical abuse when they suggest that their partners use condoms. Additionally, Dworkin and Pincu (1993) caution that AIDS may be viewed by some as a problem that affects only whites: many women of color may not perceive themselves to be at risk.

Also, appropriate terminology may not always be used in health care settings. For example, different ethnic groups may have different definitions of sexual orientation and various sexual activities. Mays and Cochran (1988) warn that poor women may be told to use condoms when they barely have enough money to buy food. Food stamps cannot be used to buy condoms, Medicaid does not cover their cost, and utilization of family planning clinics (which often offer them free) is low among women of color. While Zuckerman and Gordon (1988) suggest that nontraditional extended family arrangements may produce strong support systems, these family structures may also cause confusion regarding responsibility for the affairs of infected women and children. Thus cultural differences regarding family, intimacy, communication, sexuality, and gender roles affect wellness for women dealing with HIV/AIDS (Pizzi 1992).

Fullilove and colleagues (1990) initiated an insightful dialogue among groups of low-income African-American women in the San Francisco area. They brought the women together to talk about their sexuality, sexual practices, and feelings about AIDS. Several AIDS-related issues pervaded the discussions: the problems of male promiscuity, the power differential present within heterosexual relationships, fear of physical harm, and fear that the initiation of sex or discussion of sex will result in a woman's being labeled as a "tosser" or a poorly respected woman.

Many of these issues affect all women, but of particular importance to the low-income African-American woman are the economic constraints that exacerbate feelings of powerlessness and ineffectualness. Some women cannot demand monogamous relationships because they and their children are dependent on men for economic stability and are afraid of being cut off from them financially. Some women fear physical violence and abandonment, more prevalent in low-income communities than in middle- and upper-class communities, and therefore refrain from initiating safer sex. To them, the risk of immediate danger is greater than the chance of contracting HIV. The dangers of contracting HIV in low-income African-American communities are ever present, however, as IV drug use and drug addiction are prevalent. Some men in heterosexual relationships will have sex with women who engage in sex for drugs, which creates a high-risk situation for women, even if the woman remains monogamous. The women in Fullilove and colleagues' (1990) study who did practice safe sex emphasized the need to plan ahead and always carry a condom. It was clear, however, that only the most self-confident, assertive, and less dependent women felt comfortable demanding condom use.

Very little research has been done on the unique cultural barriers to HIV prevention experienced by Latinas. There is some evidence that Latinas, especially those living in low-income communities, experience many of the same barriers as low-income African-American women. Latin culture advocates a strong belief in family obligation and approval and male superiority. Latino men may be regarded as the decision makers, and may choose to reject condom use. Women on the other hand may be expected to suffer disappointment in silence, and to adjust to problems rather than to solve them (Pizzi 1992). Mays and Cochran (1988) propose that cultural pressures toward female naïveté among Latinas may stigmatize women who take precautions as "loose." Additionally, what is appropriate to talk about openly may prevent the dissemination of AIDS information. Sex and drugs are often considered taboo topics. Public health messages suggesting that women address sexual practices and drug use with their partners do so in ignorance of these cultural norms (Mays and Cochran 1988).

Mental health professionals must take the racial, ethnic, socioeconomic, and cultural context of minority women into consideration as they attempt to engage them in treatment. Failure to do so will likely lead to treatment failure and further alienation of the client from social service resources.

Lesbians and AIDS

Lesbians have been quite active in the fight against AIDS and the promotion of services to infected people. For many years lesbians were considered to be at little or no risk of contracting HIV because of their sexual behaviors. At this time there are no documented woman-to-woman HIV transmission cases without the presence of other recognized routes of transmission (CDC, personal communication, March 26, 1996). However, lesbians sometimes have sex with women whom are bisexual or who have had sex in the past with men. Lesbians are often lulled through misinformation into believing they are not at risk as long as they are monogamous with one person. This ignores women who might identify as lesbian, but do have sex with heterosexual or IV drug-using women, trade sex for drugs, or have been raped. Accessing this type of information will require women to engage in very intimate conversations with potential partners. Many lesbians are uncomfortable with discussing past sexual histories with new partners. Mental health professionals should encourage their lesbian clients to use latex gloves and dental dams until both partners agree to be monogamous and have been tested for HIV infection within appropriate time frames. In addition, more lesbians are deciding to have children through artificial insemination, often with sperm donated from gay men. Women considering this option should be counseled about the risks of HIV exposure associated with this method of impregnation.

Adolescent Females

Addressing female adolescents with HIV is even more complex due to the unique developmental issues and societal rules that govern them. As they struggle for autonomy and a sense of self, society sends messages encouraging them to be compliant and passive and to yield to the "superior" status of males. As a result, unique barriers are set up against their receiving information on preventing transmission and managing their infection. These infected teenagers have to ask their male partners to use a condom, a behavior that their respective peer group does not support, which requires self-efficacy—the belief that one can effect change in another individual. Many adolescent females have difficulty maintaining a healthy level of self-esteem and the degree of self-efficacy needed to carry out this task. Mental health professionals must recognize the pertinent developmental and cultural constraints that stand in the way of the adolescent female's initiating these behaviors. This includes minority females, who are currently at greatest risk (CDC 1994). In thinking about the safer-sex options listed previously, it is not difficult to imagine the conflicts many adolescent females will experience, first in discussing these behaviors with a partner, and then insisting that they engage in safer sex rather than risky, unprotected sex (Weinman et al. 1992).

Female adolescents who suspect they have been exposed to HIV are often reluctant to seek antibody testing or treatment at all due to fears that their parents or peers may discover that they are HIV positive. The limits of confidentiality with minors and their fear of exposure to friends and family may prevent them from receiving early medical treatment. This puts the mental health professional in a difficult position. The professional should focus on having the teenager tested and then facilitate the telling of the parent(s). Family therapy appears to be the most appropriate modality since the therapist will have an opportunity to empower the young woman and help dispel misbeliefs the parent(s) or other family members might have about HIV/AIDS. This requires a modification of family system interventions used by many family therapists. Family members may respond to learning that the adolescent is HIV positive in many ways—with anger, blame, grief. The mental health professional is in a good position to clarify and validate these responses while empowering the family to unite as a support system and provide the tools needed to cope with the various stages of the illness.

Commercial Sex Workers

Prostitutes or sex workers are an extremely marginalized group and difficult to reach through traditional channels. They are unlikely to approach a mental health professional voluntarily, but may come to the attention of therapists through other sources, such as drug abuse centers or hospitals. In this country sex workers are HIV infected primarily through their own IV drug use or by trading sex for drugs (Darrow 1992). Because of their drug addiction, many sex workers are unable to avoid high-risk behaviors. Sex workers have begun to form grassroots organizations to address the difficulties they face with respect to HIV infection, but there are few federal- or state-funded HIV and substance abuse prevention and treatment programs targeted specifically to them. In contrast, the United States government spends approximately $227 million annually for the arrest, prosecution, and detention of sex workers (ACT UP/NY 1990).

Commercial sex workers are a difficult population to reach and motivate to institute behavior change. When they are open to receiving assistance and engaging in self-care behaviors, mental health professionals need to be prepared to direct them to appropriate venues that will offer direct and meaningful services. If this can be accomplished, the mental health professional will have done a great deal to foster trust with the sex worker and demonstrate that positive change can be achieved.

Issues of Family and the HIV-Infected Woman

Many HIV-infected women will face the decision about whether to have a child after they have received their diagnosis. The most recent studies from the CDC suggest that expectant mothers on AZT and DDI or DDC during their pregnancy have a 50 to 75 percent chance of not having babies who are HIV positive eighteen to twenty-four months after birth (CDC 1994). Women who decide not to have children because of their HIV status are likely to undergo a period of grief or mourning for their loss. Some women will decide they will still have a child in the hope that the infant will not be infected. This may be due to societal values that place great value on a woman's role as a mother and caretaker. Moreover, women may feel a need to leave behind a legacy after their death. The mental health professional must explicitly explain the risks to the mother, but not impose her/his judgment on the woman regarding this decision. The therapist and client should fully explore the issues of who will care for her child(ren) after her illness progresses to a point where she can no longer provide direct care and whom she wants to raise them after she has died. Once identified, this person or persons should meet with both the mental health professional and the HIV/AIDS-infected woman to ensure all are in agreement with the arrangement. This process should begin before the acute onset of neurological symptoms to ensure that the woman is making well-thought-out decisions. If another parent is involved, but not in direct care of the child(ren), that parent must have input and agree to the proposed plan to spare further trauma to the child(ren) after their mother's death. Once the appropriate dialogues have taken place and future custody decisions have been made, legal documents clearly outlining the client's wishes must be made. As the disease progresses, mental health professionals should include specific grief work for all members of the woman's family, with special developmental considerations for children.

If the children are old enough to understand that their mother has HIV/AIDS, family therapy is recommended as well as individual sessions with the children. Questions should be answered clearly and sensitively, but honestly. Children will need to be reassured about the plans being made for their care and provided with a way to work through their grief. Ideally this should occur once the child knows of the mother's HIV status so that the remaining time can be most significant to the family. How much to tell the child and when will depend upon the child's cognitive capacity and developmental maturity.

Children will likely have many fears and erroneous beliefs about their mother's illness and what will happen to them after her death. The mental health professional should reassure the child that she/he is loved and will be protected. If the child is HIV infected, early medical care is critical as many infected children have neurological and cognitive impairments. The child(ren) should be told repeatedly that she/he is not responsible for his/her mother's illness. If the child is not infected, psychological treatment may need to address "survivor guilt" as well as the fears and rage often experienced at the imminent loss of the mother.

Pregnant women will need to decide whether abortion is an option. In this situation the therapist must guide the woman gently through this decision since the issues surrounding it are complex, especially for asymptomatic women. Religious, cultural, or financial constraints may eliminate abortion as an option. There is no way to identify what the HIV status of the child will be, so it is the therapist's responsibility to help the woman choose the decision that is right for her. This may present emotional difficulties for the mental health professional, especially when it is apparent that the woman has AIDS and few external resources to care for the child. In high infection areas (e.g., New York and Florida) many orphaned babies remain wards of the state and in hospitals due to the difficulty of placing HIV-positive children in foster or adoptive care.

Perhaps the most tragic scenario is the woman who already has one or more children. If the woman's HIV status is known, the children are likely to experience prejudice and avoidance from other children and their parents who fear infection somehow through casual contact. Many women with HIV lose their housing and/or insurance benefits, which jeopardizes their ability to keep their children. Low-income single mothers are in a most precarious position. If they seek help from social service agencies, they often encounter the risk of having their children placed in foster care because social service personnel may demonstrate bias and inappropriately perceive the children to be at risk in the home. The fear of losing custody of their children often prevents many HIV-infected women from receiving needed services. Care of the children is likely to be of paramount importance to most women, who will go to great lengths to maintain them in the home.

REFERENCES

Act Up/New York. *Women, AIDS, and Activism.* (1990). Boston: South End.

Brown, V. (1990). The AIDS crisis: intervention and prevention. In *Crisis intervention and prevention*, ed. H. Pruett and V. Brown, pp. 67–74. San Francisco: Jossey-Bass.

Centers for Disease Control and Prevention (CDC) (1994). *HIV/AIDS Surveillance Report*, mid-year ed., Vol. 6, No. 1. Atlanta: U.S. Department of Health and Human Services, Public Health Service.

——— (1995). *HIV/AIDS Surveillance Report* (1):10–27.

Chodorow, N. (1989). *Feminism and Psychoanalytic Theory.* New Haven: Yale University Press.

Darrow, W. W. (1992). Assessing targeted AIDS prevention in male and female prostitutes and their clients. In *Assessing AIDS Prevention*, ed. F. Paccaud, J. P. Vader, and F. Gutzwiler, pp. 215–231. Basel: Birkhauser Verlag.

Dworkin, S., and Pincu, L. (1993). Counseling in the era of AIDS. *Journal of Counseling and Development* 71:(3)275–281.

Fullilove, M. T., Fullilove, R. E., Haynes, K., and Gross, S. A. (1990). Black women and AIDS: a view towards understanding the gender rules. *Journal of Sex Research* 27:47–64.

Ickovics, J., Morrill, A., Beren, S., et al. (1994). Limited effects of HIV counseling and testing of women. *Journal of the American Medical Association* 272(6)443–448.

Jemott, J. B., Jemott, L. L., and Fong, G. T. (1992). Reductions in HIV risk associated sexual behaviors among black male adolescents: effects of an AIDS prevention intervention. *American Journal of Public Health* 82(3)372–377.

Mays, V. M., and Cochran, S. D. (1988). Issues in the perception of AIDS risk and risk reduction activities by black and Hispanic/Latina women. *American Psychologist* 43:949–957.

Pizzi, M. (1992). Women, HIV infection, and AIDS: tapestries of life, death, and empowerment. *American Journal of Occupational Therapy* 46(11)1021–1027.

Quadagno, D., Harrison, D., Wambach, K. G., et al. (1991). Women at risk for HIV. *Journal of Psychology and Human Sexuality* 4(3)97–110.

Shaw, N. (1987). AIDS: special concerns for women. In *Working with AIDS*, ed. M. Helmquist. San Francisco: University of California Regents.

Sherr, L., Petrak, J., Melvin, D., and Davey, T. (1993). Psychological trauma associated with AIDS and HIV infection in women. *Counselling Psychology Quarterly* 6(2)99–108.

Tolman, D. (1991). Adolescent girls, women, and sexuality. Discerning dilemmas of desire. In *Women, Girls, and Psychotherapy: Reframing Resistance*, ed. C. Gilligan, A. Rogers, and D. Jolman. New York: Hawthorn Press.

Weinman, M., Smith, P., and Mumford, D. (1992). A comparison between a 1986 and 1989 cohort of inner city adolescent females on knowledge, beliefs, and risk factors for AIDS. *Journal of Adolescence* 15:19–28.

Wermuth, L., Ham, J., and Robbins, R. (1991). Women don't wear condoms: AIDS risk among sexual partners of IV drug users. In *Social Relations and the AIDS Crises*, ed. J. Huber and B. E. Schneider. Newbury Park, CA: Sage.

Van De Wijgert, J. H., and Padian, N. S. (1993). Heterosexual transmission of HIV. In *AIDS and the Heterosexual Population*, ed. L. Sherr, pp. 1–19. Chur, Switzerland: Harwood Academic Publishers.

Winiarski, M. (1991). *AIDS-Related Psychotherapy*. New York: Pergamon.

Ybarra, S. (1991). Women and AIDS: implications for counseling. *Journal of Counseling and Development* 69:285–287.

Zuckerman, C., and Gordon, L. (1988). Meeting the psychosocial and legal needs of women with AIDS and their families. *New York State Journal of Medicine* 88(12):619–620.

8

The Biopsychosocial Treatment and Prevention of HIV Disease among Injection Drug Users

RALPH J. DiCLEMENTE,
SHANDOWYN L. PARKER,
NORMAN HUGGINS, AND
DENISE HORNBUCKLE

INTRODUCTION

Injection drug use has played a key role in the AIDS epidemic. Injection drug users represent the second largest group of persons to be infected with HIV in the United States and Europe. Furthermore, HIV infection within this population continues to increase in South America and Southeast Asia. In most countries, with the exception of Africa, heterosexual HIV transmission and mother-to-infant HIV transmission has most frequently been associated with injection drug use (Des Jarlais 1991).

Of those persons who have been diagnosed with HIV within the last ten years, injection drug users have shown a steady increase in infection, rising from 18 percent of the 376 cases diagnosed in 1981 to 27 percent of the 20,149 new cases reported in 1995. Statistics reported at the end of 1995 indicate that of the 470,288 persons diagnosed with AIDS, 25 percent had intravenous drug use as their only risk exposure factor. Seven percent had both IV drug use and another risk exposure factor for HIV infection (CDC 1995). IV drug use also appears to be a link between high-risk drug users and other heterosexual populations. For instance, in many perinatal transmission cases, one parent reports a history of injection drug use. The majority of the women who have been diagnosed with AIDS use or have used IV drugs, and most heterosexual transmission cases are usually a result of sexual contact with a person who has used IV drugs (Sorensen 1991).

Other factors to be considered in the issue of IV drug use and the AIDS epidemic are regional variations and ethnic and cultural issues. The prevalence of HIV infection among injection drug users in urban areas such as New Jersey and New York City ranges from 50 to 60 percent, markedly higher relative to states in the central and western regions of the country. Moreover, rates of HIV infection among African-American and Hispanic injection drug users are significantly higher than among white injection drug users (Sorensen 1991).

PSYCHOLOGICAL SEQUELAE OF HIV/AIDS: AN UNDERSTUDIED CONSEQUENCE OF DISEASE

Numerous prevention, medical, and biological issues need to be confronted when addressing the crisis of HIV/AIDS among injection drug users. Often overlooked, however, are the myriad emotional and psychosocial sequelae to HIV/AIDS. In addition to living in fear of acquiring HIV, individuals at high risk for disease acquisition encounter other sources of stress. For those who are HIV positive a key concern is social isolation and stigmatization. This compounds the marginality already confronted by many IV drug users. Moreover, for the ones who are uninfected but unable to modify the behaviors that increase their risk for HIV infection, a sense of helplessness characterized by an acquiescence that they are powerless to affect the potential threat confronting them may emerge. In general, there appears to be a continuum of HIV-related psychological problems, ranging from anxiety to full-blown immobilization, psychosis, and sometimes suicide (Ostrow 1990). These problems are typical of those that find expression during the course of HIV and AIDS.

STAGES OF HIV PROGRESSION AND ADVERSE PSYCHOLOGICAL RESPONSE

A continuum describing the progression of HIV/AIDS and its association with adverse psychological responses among IV drug users has been conceptualized by researchers and clinicians. The continuum ranges from psychological responses often associated with users' suspicions that they are infected with HIV to the actual development of AIDS. Each stage and its psychological sequelae are differentiated below.

Pre-HIV antibody testing deals with the possibility of infection. Post-HIV antibody testing concerns knowing and/or receiving seropositive test results when persons may be asymptomatic and have a stable CD-4 count. Likewise, a falling CD-4 count in which users may or may not have physical symptoms and/or prophylactic medications can be considered one of the later phases of HIV disease progression. When severe medical illness accompanies a diagnosis of AIDS, this represents the final stage in the disease process. During this stage a patient begins to experience deteriorating physical and mental functioning, followed by death.

While the stages of disease progression are based on deteriorating levels of physical functioning, it is important to note that HIV is an unpredictable and rapidly fluctuating disease condition. Thus, the heuristic provided above, while representing the experiences of many clinicians in this area, are generalizations. There are, of course, exceptions to this pattern of disease progression. Likewise, a pattern of psychological responses may be observed in correlation with the stages of disease progression. These too are subject to a wide array of human responses.

PSYCHOSOCIAL AND EMOTIONAL SEQUELAE OF HIV INFECTION

Injection drug users infected with HIV undergo numerous psychosocial and emotional problems associated with their disease. Throughout their illness they experience many emotional highs and lows among the number of psychological responses that affect their daily living. A review of the literature on HIV-related psychosocial responses shows little information on psychosocial sequelae that is specific to the stages of disease progression. It is clear, however, that to counsel and treat IV drug-using patients more effectively, clinicians need to understand the emotional problems likely to be prevalent at each stage of disease progression.

IV drug users at risk for HIV may undergo problems such as chronic tension, fearfulness, and somatic symptoms because they feel their lifestyle and behaviors may have caused them to become infected. Fear is a key component in the disease process. It is common in the earliest stages of the disease, particularly during the pre-HIV antibody testing stage when drug users are struggling with the possibility that they may be HIV infected. Fear is a significant emotional response in all stages of disease progression, but for some it can be emotionally debilitating before the individual actually learns of his/her HIV status (Miller 1990).

The post-HIV antibody testing stage or receipt of a positive HIV test result can trigger tremendous emotional upheaval. After HIV infection is identified there are two focus points for the patients. First, individuals undergo fear of the future and the course that the disease will take. Second, individuals fear the reactions of loved ones and the double stigmatization of society. HIV-positive IV drug users often carry the dual psychological burdens of feeling scorned by general society due to their drug-taking behavior and accompanying lifestyle and carrying a virus that frightens so many people. Many of these individuals view their positive HIV status as a death sentence or punishment for their lifestyles (Miller 1990). Shock and denial are important conspirators when drug users are dealing with the knowledge that they are HIV positive. Shock interferes with cognitive and behavioral functioning, thus causing problems when it comes to managing their medical treatment. IV drug users experiencing shock at the diagnosis of HIV infection may not understand all the information clinicians supply about their health or the disease process. They may withdraw, become aggressive, or may undergo cleansing or purging behavior to release anxiety over their loss of hope. Shock can be immediate, delayed, or a recurring response that may occur throughout the various stages of disease progression, especially when new adverse events (i.e., opportunistic infections) emerge (Miller 1990).

Another common psychological response to learning of an HIV-positive diagnosis is denial, a response that is twofold in nature. It functions to reduce internal stress but is problematic in that IV drug users are confused at a time when they need to be alert and informed to make important personal decisions. Because of their inability to accept their HIV status, they may seek a second opinion and request repeated HIV testing in hopes that the test results are incorrect (Miller 1990).

Anxiety related to the course of the disease, isolation, rejection, infecting others, and changes in lifestyle are all psychological responses that present themselves in HIV-infected IDUs. Anxiety may present as physical symptoms such as sweating, nausea, diarrhea, dizziness, and skin rashes. This often leads to a negative feedback loop in which these symptoms are often misinterpreted by the patient as indicators that the disease process is accelerating, often stimulating even greater levels of anxiety and rumination. It is important that clinicians be able to recognize psychological responses from neurological or physical responses associated with disease progression. Anxiety presents an additional problem for the substance abuser in that patients often revert to prescribed drugs as well as recreational drugs to manage their anxiety symptoms (Miller 1990). Anxiety can occur at any point during disease progression. It is most prominent during the early stages of the process when individuals do not know of their HIV status or have learned of their diagnosis only recently (Miller 1990).

Depression is another acute manifestation of the progression of HIV illness. Between 50 and 60 percent of methadone maintenance clients report a history of depressive disorders (Woody et al. 1991). Moreover, high levels of depressive symptoms may contribute to poor treatment outcomes and increased HIV risk (Batki et al. 1990). Often when drug-using patients reach the stage in disease progression when they are experiencing failing health—declining CD-4 counts and physical symptoms of the disease—the psychological response of depression becomes more evident. Patients are depressed as a reaction to their failing health or the inevitable decline of their health, and the accompanying physical limitations of HIV disease become more salient. Moreover, realization that a cure for AIDS is not available also leads to increased affective disturbance.

Depression alters one's relationships with friends and relatives and impacts negatively upon the individual's daily functioning and self-concept. Depression also interferes with injection drug user patients' perception of the disease as well as adaptation to and acceptance of potentially fast-changing health circumstances. Emotional and social withdrawal is commonly associated with depression among drug users at this juncture. Obstructing the adaptation process may leave the patient more fearful and self-blaming, creating more concern for the physical and mental health of the patient (Miller 1990). In addition, drug relapses are often preceded by a wish to reduce negative affect or to increase positive affect (Marlatt and Gordon 1985). A report by Gibson and colleagues (1992) found that drug users with high depression levels engaged in more frequent HIV risk behaviors, as compared to subjects with low symptom levels of depression. In addition, many IDUs are dealing with severe psychosocial stressors including poverty, homelessness or inadequate housing, medical problems, and legal difficulties.

PSYCHOLOGICAL AND EMOTIONAL SEQUELAE OF HIV INFECTION

Suicide is a potential response that is to be taken seriously. When IDU patients emotionally withdraw from their support systems, they often lose their sense of self-worth. Their lowered self-esteem may limit their ability to cope with HIV and suicidal ideation is often expressed. Suicidal ideation can occur at any time during the disease process; however, it commonly occurs after diagnosis of illness as well as during those times when the patient may experience rapid deteriorating health and feels his/her life is soon to be over (Miller 1990).

Anger, frustration, and guilt are all emotions that occur throughout the process of HIV disease. IDU patients may experience feelings of intense anger at their inability to overcome the virus. In addition, the changes in lifestyle and behavior as well as being "caught" for their behaviors are factors contributing to their anger and frustration. Guilt over having possibly exposed others to HIV and guilt over choosing behaviors that put them at risk of HIV add to the problems of coping with HIV and AIDS (Miller 1990).

PSYCHOLOGICAL INTERVENTIONS AND HIV RISK-REDUCTION

The depressive symptoms experienced by IDUs may represent a chronic difficulty that is not always alleviated by addiction treatment alone. In contrast, clients who are in treatment for alcohol dependence or cocaine dependence may initially present with high levels of depressive symptoms, but these symptoms tend to decrease significantly over the first four to eight weeks of drug treatment. Because depression is so common among IDUs, and because it appears to be related to other problem behaviors (i.e., relapse to drug use, HIV risk), it may be useful for IDUs to be screened for depression upon entry into treatment. Post-treatment assessments for affective functioning may be helpful in determining if the depressive symptoms are situational or chronic. Chronic symptoms may respond to antidepressants, psychotherapy, or a combination of these methods (Woody et al. 1982). Woody and colleagues (1983) found that clients who attended cognitive-behavioral therapy or supportive-expressive therapy, combined with methadone maintenance therapy (MMT) and drug counseling, had more positive outcomes compared with clients who received only MMT and drug counseling.

NEUROPSYCHIATRIC MANIFESTATIONS OF HIV INFECTION

Neuropsychiatric disorders are common in HIV infection. Patients show signs of neuropsychiatric disorders across the spectrum of HIV disease: from early HIV infection when few or no symptoms are present to the time one develops full-blown AIDS when a number of complications have arisen. Neuropsychiatric and psychosocial factors need to be addressed as a unit because both are of considerable importance in HIV infection. When abnormal emotional and mental disturbances become issues in the progression of HIV, clinicians need to consider the potential neuropsychiatric component of the problems before determining that psychosocial complications are the sole reason for the patient's problems (Fernandez and Levy 1990).

HIV plays havoc on the central nervous system. Many patients present with cognitive impairment, psychosis, language and movement disorders, delirium, and depression during various stages of the disease process (Fernandez and Levy 1990). AIDS dementia complex is an affliction that impairs brain function, markedly diminishing the quality of remaining life in AIDS patients. It slows intellectual processing, decreases ability to concentrate, and reduces the patient to a shell of his/her former self (Auerbach et al. 1994). Neuropsychiatric disorders are important issues of concern at all phases of illness but become of extreme importance during the final stage of AIDS when decisions about life-sustaining treatment need to be addressed such as consent for medical services and developing living wills for carrying out a person's final wishes in the eventuality of death. Often during this phase, mental functioning is very limited and clinicians must play a role in assessing the mental competence of the patient (Ostrow 1990).

As described previously, HIV causes a great deal of psychosocial and neuropsychiatric complications without the added complications of substance abuse. However, in combination, both illnesses can present a multitude of complications and adverse consequences. A high prevalence of psychosocial disorders— anxiety, personality disorders, and depression—already exists among injection drug users. Moreover, depression was identified as a predictive factor associated with risk-taking behavior among intravenous drug users. Also, psychiatric disorders have been identified as one factor in why substance abusers do not comply with prescribed medical care for their HIV infection. Clearly, in disentangling the adverse psychological responses attributable to HIV disease and intravenous drug use, it is important to study the co-morbidity of the two diseases. Studies to examine risk-taking tendencies and avoidance of medical treatment using mental health determinants will help in the development of strategies to enhance follow-up care. Furthermore, addressing the issues jointly helps clinicians and researchers to recognize and understand the importance of pursuing research that combines mental health services, drug abuse treatment, and medical care for HIV infection (Auerbach et al. 1994).

STRATEGIES FOR COPING WITH HIV INFECTION

After an IDU learns that he/she is HIV positive, many seem to have difficulty contending with the numerous emotions and lifestyle changes HIV engenders. It is important that IDUs learn to employ coping strategies and social support as a means of surviving the adverse psychological changes that occur and are associated with the various stages of HIV disease progression. Cognitive restructuring, thought stopping, and establishing situations that allow the patient to experience feelings of self-efficacy and self-control are the types of strategies that appear to promote enhanced psychological well-being throughout the course of HIV infection (Auerbach et al. 1994).

To help moderate the anxiety that often accompanies a recent diagnosis of HIV infection or AIDS, the IDU is provided with appropriate and current information regarding the virus (i.e., virology and clinical course, infectiousness, and treatment protocols). Emphasizing the confidential nature of the therapeutic relationship and focusing upon establishing a supportive alliance with the IDU are essential activities for the professional working with this population. If the IDU requires a period of withdrawal from the addictive drug, the professional should be attentive to the development of depression within the patient. For many IDUs, undergoing the process of physical and psychological withdrawal from their addictive drug along with the realization that he/she is impacted by HIV is emotionally overwhelming. Suicidal ideation is not uncommon and should be assessed periodically. The establishment of a support system for the IDU is imperative at this time (Miller 1990). Assisting the IDU in creating a network of support (i.e., family, nondrug-abusing friends, mental health or drug counseling professionals, medical management team, clergy, and so on) is crucial to assisting the IDU in maintaining a sense of hope through-out the course of HIV disease (Auerbach et al. 1994).

When dealing with the final stages of life, questions may arise as to the mental capacity of the IDU patient. At a time when decisions are to be made about medical concerns and legal issues such as living wills, it is imperative that clinicians assess the competence of a patient to give informed consent (Ostrow 1990). To avoid situations where the patient is not able to give informed consent, patients should be informed early in the disease process about the potential for developing cognitive impairments so that they can make arrangements to have a friend or loved one have power of attorney to make important decisions for the well-being of the patient.

DEATH AND DYING AND THE SUBSTANCE ABUSER

In dealing with any terminal illness, death and dying are issues that are difficult but must be addressed. In the case of AIDS, the issue is no different but can be more difficult to handle, especially because the illness greatly affects a younger population (25–39-year-old age group). This population often feels that life is endless; therefore, addressing thoughts of death is undesirable and is often avoided. Substance abusers who are accustomed to dealing with death because of a lifestyle that puts them in the path of harm many times—attributable to violence, overdose, and contaminated drugs—see death as a means of "paying their dues." They may not understand the importance of making final arrangements or resolving the unfinished areas of their lives as do many persons who are dying with AIDS and are not substance abusers (Ottomanelli 1992).

THE ROLE OF SUBSTANCE ABUSE TREATMENT

Substance abuse treatment is one of the most effective methods for reducing the spread of HIV among hard-core drug users and their sex partners. Participation in treatment, even for HIV-positive substance abusers, decreases the chance of HIV transmission and reduces the risk of exposure to variants of HIV. Effective treatment can reduce and/or eliminate needle use and provide a pathway to education on related risk behaviors.

Although treatment for drug dependence is considered the optimal intervention for IDUs, other HIV prevention strategies must be used for those who are not in treatment and for those for whom treatment is not totally effective. For every active IDU in treatment, six are not. Analysis of past National Institute of Drug Abuse projects found that at first contact, 41 percent of IDUs had never been in treatment despite an average substance abuse history of eleven years. The significant risk to the IDU, their sex partners, and children indicates a continuing need to reach this population and enhance their entry into treatment. In addition, the seropositive IDU needs strategies to slow the progression of AIDS illnesses and may benefit from the network of services that extend from treatment centers. Realistically, there will remain a significant portion of substance abusers who cannot or will not enter substance abuse treatment but who can and will alter risk behaviors associated with HIV transmission if the strategy is appropriate to their needs. Interventions should take into account gender, race/ethnicity, sexual orientation, and/or risk behaviors as well as the social context in which the individual behaviors occur. With sensitive intervention, many IDUs can make positive behavior changes although a large percentage may require additional assistance to maintain their lower risk profiles.

Knowledge of the individual IDU's serostatus appears to have a positive moderating effect on risk behavior. This indicates that there is a critical need to identify the presence of HIV at the earliest opportunity through confidential testing and counseling programs. Effective counseling may facilitate the IDU's access to medical treatment and can support the clinical management of AIDS illness by encouraging the IDU to keep clinic appointments and to comply with any identified medical regimen. In addition to HIV counseling and testing of hard-core drug users, one aspect of integrated client services can involve partner notification efforts to provide counseling and testing services to a hidden at-risk population. If sex and/or needle-sharing partners are found to be seropositive they can also receive early intervention for HIV and transmission of the virus could be interrupted.

There is a need to improve strategies for assisting the active IDU in the reduction of HIV risk behaviors. Such efforts need to reflect culturally relevant information for the population being served and include the two most effective strategies identified to date, that is, early, individualized testing and counseling services and access to substance abuse treatment. Injection drug use is only one of a constellation of risk behaviors which must be addressed.

AIDS RISK REDUCTION FOR IV DRUG USERS

Due to the HIV–substance-use connection, many drug abuse treatment programs need to provide programs aimed at reducing substance abuser's risk for acquiring HIV, particularly among high-risk injection drug users. Risk-reduction programs need to utilize cost-effective strategies aimed at reaching large groups of drug users, and more importantly, programs must be practical to have any significant impact on this population. Widespread distribution of pamphlets is helpful but is not sufficient to motivate substance abusers to modify high-risk behaviors (Gibson and Lovelle-Drache 1991). Little literature exists addressing psychosocial variables of substance abuse-related behaviors and how they are correlated with risk behaviors. There is also a dearth of literature available for understanding the role that different psychosocial variables play at various stages in the substance abuser's process of changing risk behaviors (Gibson et al. 1991). Moreover, there are few psychosocial models of risk reduction that have been specifically developed for this high-risk population. One model, the AIDS Risk Reduction Model, may be appropriate for developing behavior modification interventions for injecting drug users.

AIDS RISK REDUCTION MODEL: APPLICABILITY TO INJECTION DRUG USERS

A three-stage model, the AIDS Risk Reduction Model (ARRM), has been proposed by Catania and his colleagues (1990) to address people's efforts to change sexual behavior. The model is based on sexual behavior changes as they pertain to risk of HIV infection, but with a few modifications it can be equally applicable to HIV-related injection drug use behaviors.

The ARRM suggests that behavior change is attained by consecutive stages of labeling, commitment, and action. Labeling deals with an individual's becoming educated on the transmission of AIDS and aware of his/her own susceptibility to the disease. Knowledge of their enhanced susceptibility promotes individuals to think about their behaviors and how those behaviors put them at risk of HIV. Upon advancing to stage two, the commitment stage, an individual finds effective means of reducing risk; this is commonly referred to as *response efficacy*. Also, a part of commitment involves *self-efficacy*, which deals with one's perception of his/her ability to change. Through the last stage, enactment, a person moves closer to the goal of change by means of either self-help or help from others (Gibson and Lovelle-Drache 1991).

Knowledge is a part of labeling in that a drug user learns about HIV transmission and facts concerning injection drug use so that assessing risk is confronted on a personal level. Susceptibility is important in the earlier stages of change because drug users now perceive that their behaviors may put them at risk.

Response efficacy is how one views the effectiveness of health-promoting or HIV-preventive practices that are recommended by health personnel. After acknowledging problems with behavior, the next step for the drug user is to make a commitment to reduce risk behaviors. For example, drug users may agree to "shoot up" only at home where they can keep sterile needles accessible or have access to bleach and water to clean their drug equipment.

Self-efficacy is a necessary component to the model. Drug users have to believe they have the ability to change behaviors and remain committed to their changes. Self-efficacy becomes important when drug users are faced with situations where they may be tempted to perform risky behaviors regardless of the consequences to their health. Communication skills and social support are combined in stage three of the model. The ability to discuss the behaviors in question will be a key component in the enactment stage. In like manner, social support is instrumental in that drug users have a link to someone when they need assistance in continuing their progress in making permanent behavioral changes (Gibson et al. 1991).

To make permanent changes in behavior, risk-reduction strategies must focus on the different stages of change that the drug user will undergo. Outreach campaigns that focus on bombarding drug users with pamphlets are primarily important to alert IDUs of the threat of HIV and the behaviors that place them at risk for infection; however, they alone cannot motivate drug users to change their behavior. Behavior change strategies that include components that promote self-efficacy and response efficacy are the important second-level elements that are necessary to foster potentially lifesaving alterations in cognition and behavior within this population.

STRUCTURAL CHANGES IN PROVIDING DRUG USERS WITH MEDICAL CARE FOR HIV DISEASE

To a large extent, this chapter has focused primarily on the psychological responses of drug users at different stages of HIV disease progression and strategies for modifying high-risk behaviors among drug users. However, of considerable importance to ameliorating these adverse psychological responses and promoting the adoption and maintenance of HIV-preventive behaviors are structural changes within the drug treatment system itself.

Drug treatment programs have attempted to study HIV infection of intravenous drug users by examining the epidemiology of HIV infection and injection drug use. Few treatment programs have instituted systematic approaches to address the issue of prevention of HIV transmission among injection drug users. Moreover, numerous drug treatment programs have chosen not to deal with the problem of HIV/AIDS altogether, opting to transfer clients out of their programs or deny admission into treatment programs based on a positive HIV test result (Des Jarlais 1991).

Drug abuse treatment programs faced with the AIDS epidemic can expand to include HIV-related medical services. Methadone treatment programs, in particular, offer an excellent opportunity for providing medical care for several reasons. Drug abusers who may distrust traditional medical systems and who may not want to attend AIDS clinics for fear of stigmatization can be medically treated at the same sites where they receive methadone treatment. Finally, methadone programs have daily contact with patients who have chaotic lifestyles and are often erratic in their compliance with medical regimens. On-site medical care can provide flexibility by allowing patients to be seen on a "drop in" basis rather than by appointment. This may be particularly helpful for female IDUs who find it difficult to arrange child care. In addition, staff who dispense methadone can also dispense other medications, as well as monitor compliance and follow-up (Roehrich et al. 1994).

Examples of methadone programs that have implemented on-site medical services can be found in New York City and San Francisco, two areas severely impacted by the AIDS epidemic. These programs now provide primary medical care for patients with, or at high-risk for, HIV infection (Batki et al. 1990, Selwyn et al. 1989). The medical care includes routine admission and annual physical examinations required in all methadone programs, PAP tests for women, treatment for acute HIV-related illness and prophylactic regimens, as well as referrals and consultation with specialized AIDS clinics.

Increasing compliance with anti-retroviral treatments, such as Zidovudine (AZT), may be especially urgent. AZT can delay progression of HIV disease and improve quality of life (Fischel et al. 1991, Volberding et al. 1990). However, because of its short half-life, AZT is prescribed as multiple daily doses. Moreover, AZT has severe side effects. Thus, it may be particularly difficult for patients to adhere to their prescribed medical treatment regimens. In addition, AZT is offered as often but is accepted *less* often by IDUs compared to HIV-infected patients in other risk groups (Broers et al. 1992). Significantly lower rates of AZT compliance have been noted among patients with a history of IDU (Fischl 1991, Samet et al. 1992); consequently, compliance with AZT may be increased by having one of the daily doses administered at methadone clinics.

On-site medical care in methadone programs can also monitor for other HIV-related diseases such as Pneumocystis carinii pneumonia (PCP) and tuberculosis (TB), as well as provide prophylactic medications for these diseases. TB, for example, is increasingly prevalent in the United States. New infections are especially common among certain high-risk groups including people with HIV disease, IDUs, and racial or ethnic minority groups. Medical treatment of tuberculin skin test positive (PPD+) patients currently consists of a standard chemoprophylaxis regimen such as six months of isoniazid or rifampin. Compliance with TB chemoprophylaxis is typically poor among IDUs. Poor compliance can lead to no treatment or incomplete treatment, both of which result in the failure to prevent TB. Active TB can rapidly spread among IDUs, particularly in persons who are HIV infected.

Methadone programs with on-site medical care can also more readily monitor the complex regimens of multiple medications and the interactions of pharmacologic treatments. A classic example is a drug such as rifampin that induces liver enzymes and may reduce the activity of several drugs, including methadone and dapsone (Amodio-Groton and Currier 1992). In order to enhance compliance, treatment providers must appreciate the patients' difficulty in adhering to complex pharmaceutical regimens that may potentially include unpleasant side effects; patients' concerns must be addressed in a prompt and direct manner. Providing on-site medical care is an effective way of providing secondary prevention of common life-threatening and contagious disorders and may reduce the morbidity and cost associated with HIV disease.

*   *   *

AIDS has become a medical and public health problem among drug abusers. Understanding the impact of HIV disease and the different stages of disease progression on drug users' psychological responses and their needs for medical care is critical to tailoring psychological counseling and medical services to address those needs. In addition, it appears that negative psychological states (i.e., depression) may facilitate increased high-risk behavior and poor treatment outcomes. Clearly, further studies utilizing prospective research designs are necessary to quantify the prevalence of adverse psychological responses and the magnitude of their association with increased risk-taking behavior, and to examine effective strategies for enhancing drug users' coping skills and adaptive capacity.

In the absence of an effective treatment or prophylactic vaccine, prevention of HIV infection is the most powerful weapon to reduce the burden of disease impact on drug users. And, while there have been encouraging changes in HIV-related sexual and drug behaviors among this population, many continue to be at risk for HIV infection. Until prevention efforts are more effective at promoting risk reduction, drug users will continue to become infected with HIV. Consequently, continued effort must be directed at understanding and minimizing the psychological and physiological impact of HIV infection on drug users.

REFERENCES

Amodio-Groton, M., and Currier, J. (1992). HIV drug interactions. *AIDS Clinical Care* 4:25–29.

Auerbach, J., Wypijewska, C., and Brodie, H. K., eds. (1994). Disease progression and intervention, pp. 124–153. In *AIDS and Behavior.* Washington, DC: National Academy Press.

Batki, S. L., Sorensen, J. L., Gibson, D. R., and Maude-Griffin, P. (1990). HIV-infected IV drug users in methadone treatment: outcome and psychological correlates—a preliminary report. *Problems of Drug Dependence, 1989*, ed. L. S. Harris, DHHS Publication No. ADM 90–1663, pp. 405–406. Rockville, MD: NIDA.

Broers, B., Hirschel, B., Gabriel V., and Morabia A. (1992). *Compliance of drug users with Zidovudine treatment.* Poster presented at the VII International Conference on AIDS, Amsterdam, Netherlands, July.

Catania, J. A., Kegeles, S., and Coates, T. J. (1990). Towards an understanding of risk behavior: an AIDS risk reduction model (ARRM). *Health Education Quarterly* 17:53–72.

Centers for Disease Control and Prevention (CDC) (1995). *HIV/AIDS Surveillance Report, 1995* 7(1):11–21.

Des Jarlais, D. (1991). Foreword. In *Preventing AIDS in Drug Users and Their Sexual Partners*, by J. Sorensen et al., pp. xi–xiv. New York: Guilford.

Fernandez, F., and Levy, J. (1990). Diagnosis and management of HIV primary dementia. In *Behavioral Aspects of AIDS*, ed. D. G. Ostrow, pp. 235–246.

Fischl, M. A., Parker, C. B., Pettinelli, C., Wulfsohn, M., et al. (1991). A randomized controlled trial of a reduced daily dose of Zidovudine in patients with the acquired immunodeficiency syndrome. *New England Journal of Medicine* 323:1009–1014.

Gibson, D., and Lovelle-Drache, J. (1991). Individual counseling. In *Preventing AIDS in Drug Users and Their Sexual Partners*, ed. J. Sorensen et al., pp. 116–129. New York: Guilford.

Gibson, D., Catania, J., and Peterson, J. (1991). Theoretical background. In *Preventing AIDS in Drug Users and Their Sexual Partners*, ed. J. Sorensen, L. A. Wermuth, D. R. Gibson, K. Choi, et al., pp. 62–74. New York: Guilford.

Gibson, D., Lovelle-Drache, J., Young, M., and Chesney, M. (1992). *HIV risk linked to psychopathology in IV drug users.* Paper presented at the VIII International Conference on AIDS, Amsterdam, Netherlands, July.

Marlatt, G. A., and Gordon, J. R. (1985). *Relapse Prevention.* New York: Guilford.

Miller, D. (1990). Diagnosis and treatment of acute psychological problems related to HIV infection and disease. In *Behavorial Aspects of AIDS*, ed. D. G. Ostrow, pp. 187–206. New York: Plenum.

Ostrow, D. (1990). Psychiatric aspects of AIDS: an overview. In *Behavioral Aspects of AIDS*, ed. D. G. Ostrow, pp. 9–18. New York: Plenum.

Ottomanelli, G. (1992). *HIV Infection and Intravenous Drug Use.* Westport, CT: Praeger.

Roehrich, L., Wall, T. L., and Sorensen, J. L. (1994). Behavioral interventions for in-treatment injection drug users. In *Preventing AIDS: Theories and Methods of Behavioral Interventions*, ed. R. J. DiClemente and J. Peterson, pp. 189–203. New York, NY: Plenum.

Samet, J. H., Libman, H., Steger, K. A., Dhawan, R. K., et al. (1992). Compliance with Zidovudine therapy in patients infected wtih human immunodeficiency virus, type I: a cross-sectional study in a municipal hospital clinic. *The American Journal of Medicine* 92:495–502.

Selwyn, P. A., Feingold, A. R., Iezza, A., Satyadeo, M., et al. (1989). Primary care for patients with human immunodeficiency virus (HIV) infection in a methadone maintenance treatment program. *Annals of Internal Medicine* 110:761–763.

Sorensen, J. L. (1991). Introduction: the AIDS-drug connection. In *Preventing AIDS in Drug Users and Their Sexual Partners*, ed. J. L. Sorensen, L. A. Wermuth, D. R. Gibson, K. Choi, et al. pp. 3–17. New York, NY: Guilford.

Volberding, P. A., Lagakos, S. W., Koch, M. A., Pettinelli, C., et al. (1990). Zidovudine in asymptomatic human immunodeficiency virus infection: a controlled trial in persons with fewer than 500 CD4-positive cells per cubic millimeter. *New England Journal of Medicine* 322:941–949.

Woody, G. E., Luborsky, L., McLellan, A. T., O'Brien, C. P., et al. (1983). Psychotherapy for opiate addicts. *Archives of General Psychiatry* 40:639–645.

Woody, G. E., McLellan, A. T., O'Brien, C. P., and Luborsky, L. (1991). Addressing psychiatric comorbidity. In *Improving Drug Abuse Treatment*, ed. R. Pickens, C. Leukefeld, and C. Schuster, pp. 152–166. DHHS Publication No. ADM 91–1754. Rockville, MD: NIDA.

Woody, G. E., O'Brien, C. P., McLellan, A. T., Marcovici, M., et al. (1982). The use of antidepressants with methadone in depressed maintenance patients. *Annals of the New York Academy of Science* 398:120–127.

Index